Advance Praise

"*Body rites* is an incredibly grounding, sensitive, and info
who've experienced sexual assault feel reconnected to their ~~bodies. dr. young~~ does a masterful job of fostering a sense of safety and warmth as she walks beside readers on the journey of healing. The book breaks down scientific and psychological terms in accessible and
relevant ways, and is a radical and needed departure from other texts in this space. Many
will be able to see themselves and be helped by her offering."

—**Joy Harden Bradford, PhD**, licensed psychologist, founder of
Therapy for Black Girls, and author of *Sisterhood Heals*

"As I read just the first few pages of this masterpiece, I felt a swirling in my stomach—the
kind that brings you a genuine sense of excitement and awe as you know you are about to curl
up with something that is going to change both your life and the world. I organically rested
a palm on my belly and heart to be present with this deeply embodied experience. dr shena
is a poet and a healer, and in *body rites* she offers the gift of her breathtaking wisdom that is
filled with the magic, light, and soothing balm only she can provide.

The illustrations are ethereal, and they beautifully affirm the holistic medicine dr. shena
shares. In this mind, body, and spirit journey of ritual, affirmation, remembrance, journaling,
embodiment, breathwork, and nervous system care, she reminds readers that they are inherently whole. A beloved spirit guide and a truly one-of-a-kind resource, may Black survivors of
sexual trauma all over the world be held, seen, and cherished with this medicine. Profoundly
healing and infused with the utmost love, care, intention from tender and deep lived experience, you will not be the same person after this journey unfolds."

—**Zahabiyah Yamasaki, MEd**, RYT, author of *Trauma-Informed Yoga for Survivors of
Sexual Assault* and *Trauma-Informed Yoga Affirmation Card Deck*

"*Body rites* is a loving invitation to return to the old technologies of ancient global cultures
to heal and bring forth new strength. By tapping into the epic memory of the body, survivors can rewrite their stories, not only the moments of harm but also what they have been
socialized to believe about themselves. *body rites* meets survivors where they are, skillfully
blending science-backed, trauma-informed best practices, spirituality, and tradition. shena
writes with patience, warmth, expertise, and courage; it is clear that each of the words and
chosen images are glimpses of shena's embodied practice offered as a gift to other survivors.
Many survivors will immediately see themselves in these pages of *body rites*, while others
will find themselves."

—**Shesheena A. Bray, MSEd**, NCC, owner of Going Inward Wellness, LLC,
and program director of me too. International

body rites

body rites

a holistic healing and embodiment
workbook for Black survivors
of sexual trauma

shena j young

foreword by Aishah Shahidah Simmons
illustrations by shyma el sayed

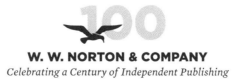

W. W. NORTON & COMPANY
Celebrating a Century of Independent Publishing

"Window of Tolerance" figure adapted from TRAUMA AND THE BODY: A SENSO-RIMOTOR APPROACH TO PSYCHOTHERAPY by Pat Ogden, Kenkuni Minton, Clare Pain. Copyright © 2006 by Pat Ogden. Copyright © 2006 by W. W. Norton & Company, Inc. Used by permission of W. W. Norton & Company, Inc.

Illustrations by shyma el sayed

For information about permission to reproduce selections from this book, write to Permissions, W. W. Norton & Company, Inc., 500 Fifth Avenue, New York, NY 10110

For information about special discounts for bulk purchases, please contact W. W. Norton Special Sales at specialsales@wwnorton.com or 800-233-4830

Manufacturing by Versa Press
Book design by Janay Frazier
Production manager: Gwen Cullen

ISBN: 978-1-324-01983-1 (pbk)

W. W. Norton & Company, Inc., 500 Fifth Avenue, New York, NY 10110
www.wwnorton.com

W. W. Norton & Company Ltd., 15 Carlisle Street, London W1D 3BS

1 2 3 4 5 6 7 8 9 0

I believe you.

you know who you are.

I'm sorry I couldn't protect you.

I am here with you, on all sides of you, and on your healing journey, for however long it takes . . .

this is OUR cauldron.
let your touch and breath on these pages
be the fire underneath
the spirit waters boiling inside
the smoke carrying your healing stories beyond

this is for survivors of sexual assault in all forms,
silently screaming in Black bodies
living beside themselves
toning their porousness
fervently returning to themselves, discovering joy
alchemizing generations of pain in their dna
making healing choices that reach forward and backward
this is for those who insist on knowing their bodies as home.

I love you, truly.

CONTENTS

prayer |

may every moment in healing happen underneath the gaze and
in the embrace of your ancestors.
may they be venerated by your choices to do what they couldn't.
may your collective body be soft and fierce, inevitably.

BREATHE IN FROM YOUR ROOT CHAKRA

Welcome, Dear One! You have entered a Black woman, femme, and nonbinary survivor–centered sanctuary, envisioned and created by my sister–survivor–friend, dr. shena j young,* a Black woman, licensed body-centered psychologist–healer, artist, and Iyalorisa.

OUR ORIGIN STORY (THE ABBREVIATED VERSION)

In the fall of 2020, during a session with DaRa Elebe Williams, my trauma-informed psycho-therapist, one of my Dharma teachers, and beloved big sister–friend, asked me if I would be interested in exploring the possibility of writing the foreword to a groundbreaking workbook for Black survivors written by a Black woman psychologist. Almost without hesitation, I enthusiastically said, "Yes." DaRa has decades of expertise working at the intersections of healing intergenerational trauma, spiritual practice, and social justice. Her guiding support has been invaluable on my journey. I knew I wanted to be involved if DaRa extended an opportunity for me to be included in a project whose vision and goal is to support Black survivors. Several weeks later, DaRa connected me with shena. While we've been in each other's orbits, our paths never intersected until DaRa brought us together.

Have you ever met someone for the first time, yet felt like you knew them for a long time? That was the feeling I experienced during my first Zoom conversation with shena. For a couple of hours, our conversation flowed like warm maple syrup over gluten-free blue-berry banana waffles. We traversed so much ground, including our survivor experiences, our sacred practices and rituals that we utilize to heal the physical, emotional, spiritual, and psychic places we've traveled on our healing journeys, our favorite foods and music, and our commitment to creating work that's in service to the wellness and healing of dias-poric Black survivors. When shena talked about her literary baby *body rites: a holistic heal-ing and embodiment workbook for Black survivors of sexual trauma*, I was in awe of her vision and process. I must share that her spoken words about her book were so profound that I had a bodily response to just hearing about it, without reading one word or viewing one image. I experienced butterflies in my stomach and warm sensations throughout my body. I wanted to enter the *body rites* sanctuary. I was and will forever be honored that her invitation to write the foreword allowed me to *BE* with the workbook for months before it was released to the world. This was a sacred gift and auspicious responsibility. By the end of our conversation, I was sure our ancestors ordained our connection, and they chose our beloved big sister–friend–guide DaRa to serve as the liaison. Àṣẹ.

---

* I use dr. shena and shena interchangeably with love.

MY PAST IS PROLOGUE

Twenty-nine years ago, in 1994, I embarked on a 12-year journey to write, direct, and produce the groundbreaking film *NO! The Rape Documentary* (2006) about intra-racial sexual violence, healing, and accountability in Black communities. At that time, I named that I was a survivor of childhood and young adult rape, but I didn't go into many details. I said, "I'm an incest and rape survivor." I was in therapy with Dr. Clara Whaley-Perkins, a Black woman and licensed clinical psychologist. Those sessions were not only a lifeline, but supported me from 1992–2020. In the mid-1990s, I vividly remember having intense research and development conversations with Dr. Tamara L. Xavier, my beloved sister–friend who is a coproducer and the director of the choreography of *NO! The Rape Documentary*. She pushed me to include dance in the film; initially, it was an uphill battle for her. Tamara was among the first to teach me that the body has memory. We can't just talk our way out of trauma. We have to move the trauma through and out of our bodies. I am grateful for Tamara's insistence and persistence, which led to the inclusion of dance in *NO! The Rape Documentary*.

TRANSPARENCY

Even with my herstory I just shared about learning that we must move the trauma through and out of our bodies, I still wanted to engage with *body rites: a holistic healing and embodiment workbook for Black survivors of sexual trauma* from a purely theoretical, "heady" stance. I wanted to barrel through it so I could write the foreword.

I didn't want to be in my body. I tried to hide in my head. Yet, I know the "body keeps the score" (van der Kolk, 2014).

When I opened both my mind and my body to dr. shena's *body rites*, and viewed the illustrations for several weeks, I wept.

I wept because I was grateful for this offering. I wept because I wholeheartedly wished it existed 30 years ago when I was in the early stages of the sexual trauma-healing journey during my mid-20s.

Dr. shena's guiding words, rituals, incantations, journal prompts, and prayers called me to move from my head down to my neck, shoulders, arms, wrists, hands, fingers, chest, heart, breasts, stomach, intestines, uterus, ovaries, vagina, buttocks, thighs, knees, legs, ankles, feet, and toes. I'm a Buddhist whose two decades of experience practicing vipassana meditation on long-term residential retreats and daily "sitting" (meditation) practices is a grounding anchor. dr. shena's invitational call in *body rites* deepened these practices that support my healing. The workbook provided a salve for some survivor wounds that decades upon decades later are still festering beneath the surface. Her language made me feel like I had extended, private sessions with her and my most intimate self. I felt seen, cared for, nurtured, and supported by dr. shena, but most importantly, by myself.

My buckets of tears were a healing release of so much that was stored in my body, from being molested as a little girl and raped as a college-aged woman. My engagement with *body rites* was a cleansing. Trauma is multilayered and intergenerational. *Body rites* is a workbook that I will return to again and probably again. It's not a one-and-done experience for me. It's one of those companions that is a new, essential part of my healing toolbox.

THE UNBROKEN CIRCLE

Body rites join a small, literary chorus of pioneering Black survivor authored and centered nonfiction books that, unlike *body rites*, are not workbooks, but serve as guides for Black survivors on our healing journeys. These include but are not limited to Dr. Charlotte Pierce-Baker's, *Surviving the Silence: Black Women's Stories of Rape* (Norton, 1998), Lori S. Robinson's *I Will Survive: The African-American Guide to Healing from Sexual Assault and Abuse* (Seal Press, 2003), and *No Secrets No Lies: How Black Families Can Heal from Sexual Abuse* (Harmony/Rodale, 2005).

THE TIME IS NOW

Continuing and expanding upon the work that precedes her own, dr. shena womanifested *body rites*, a groundbreaking, beautiful, interactive workbook that places Black women, femmes, and nonbinary survivors, in our diversity, at the center. We're not marginalized as a sidebar, a small section we must peruse through the index to find, or an afterthought. We are dr. shena's unwavering, razor-sharp focus.

Body rites is a sacred gift whose trauma-informed healing focus is African ancestral, spiritual, somatic, emotional, and mental. dr. shena invites us to choose to heal and be engaged participants in our healing. Her invitational call reminds us that healing from sexual trauma is not a spectatorial, nor solely a theoretical process. Healing is fully embodied, and dr. shena provides the resources to support our journeys.

For many Black survivors, an integral part of our embodiment is for the intersection of our racial, gender, and sexual identities to be witnessed and affirmed.

We do not have to choose which identity to focus on when journeying through and with *body rites*. We are whole precisely because of our multiple identities embodied into one. dr. shena's words are our compassionate and supportive witness, and shyma el sayed's illustrations reflect our beauty and power through different sizes, complexions, and physical abilities. This is the Black survivor magic that dr. shena conjured.

This workbook is not a one-sitting read. Of course, you can do that if you desire. It's all about choices, after all. However, *body rites* is an experience where you have to do the work to move with and through the trauma. dr. shena provides a solid foundation that includes a wealth of information about trauma and how our bodies react, including shutting down in response. Equally important, she also encourages us to listen to the wisdom of our bodies and spirits. dr. shena offers self-guided contemplative assignments, journal prompts, yoga, and other movement practices, recipes for teas and tinctures, and sacred rituals geared to dislodge the often intergenerational trauma stored in our bodies and psyches to support deep, cellular healing which is multilayered, and often requires a slow, deliberate, and intentional journey. This is intuitional work. It is your road map to your healing path.

THE CONTINUUM

In the opening of her award-winning 1980 novel, *The Salt Eaters*, the late Black feminist writer, one of my teachers, and elder sister–friend Toni Cade Bambara asked a timeless prophetic question, "Are you sure, sweetheart, you want to be well? . . . Just so's you're sure, sweetheart, and ready to be healed, cause wholeness is no trifling matter. A lot of weight when you're well." Over forty years later, dr. shena young's *body rites* is a contemporary literary affirmation of Bambara's words. Like Bambara, shena reminds us that being well is a lot of work, a huge responsibility, and a profound gift. She calls on us to remember that which is ancestral and provides roadmaps and other accompanying tools to support the healing pathway after trauma.

I remember how Toni Cade Bambara frequently told students and friends, "It's the community you want to name you and claim you . . . as sista, daughter, mother, auntie, friend." She always reminded us that we didn't want to be beholden to the corporate entities focused on our annihilation. Instead, we want to create cultural work that speaks directly to our Black communities, usually resulting in a shift from the Eurocentric gaze. Despite not meeting Toni Cade Bambara in person, shena answers Toni's (now) ancestral call for accountability to Black communities. I unequivocally believe *body rites* is part of the tradition Toni spoke of continuously. shena boldly, compassionately, and unapologetically speaks directly to Black women, femmes, and nonbinary survivors. All are welcome, and we are the center.

SANKOFA

Sankofa is the mythical bird of the Akan people in Ghana. Its head turned backward, facing the past, its feet turned forward to face the future, and its body centered in the present moment. *Body rites* is past, present, and future. It emphasizes the here and now while connecting readers to their past and supporting them in envisioning their future. For me, this is the powerful African, Indigenous, and ancestral wisdom that informs the continuum of which *body rites* is a part.

I rejoice, dr. shena. I bow deep in honor of your work that will transform countless lives. Exhale.

Aishah Shahidah Simmons, survivor–healer,
trauma-informed mindfulness meditation teacher,
producer, writer, and director of *NO! The Rape Documentary* (2006), and
editor of *love WITH Accountability: Digging Up the Root of Child Sexual Abuse* (AK Press, 2019)
June 2023

References

Bambara, T. C. (1980). *The salt eaters*. Random House.

van der Kolk, B. (2014). *The body keeps the score*. Penguin.

foreword

Intro & Welcome |

dear beloved, can I call you that? I mean it as an offering of deep endearment.

(be)loved. It is also an invitation. A beckoning to return to what is true.

I am elated that you are here, that you were led here, that you are opening to healing here.

It is my honor to be your guide. My name is dr. shena young; my beloveds call me dr. shena. I am a body centered and holistic psychologist–healer, trauma-informed educator, consultant, yoga teacher, and survivor of many things. I created this healing space, *body rites*, for you, for yours, for all of us. I wish I could tell you when this all began, when I first started collecting and intuiting the healing wisdom and tools that will follow. I value knowing the inception of power, of knowing how a story began, but I am learning that time does not like to be contained or understood. It prefers to beat wildly, to pass freely. I am learning that healing and time are conjoined, that they hold onto their truths while moving together.

> *healing is in process (v.)*
> *it is a process (n.)*
> *it is something to own.*
> *it is infinite—*
> *above & beyond.*
> *it is mine & yours & ours.*
> *it is time.*

I hope you remember these truths as you move in and out and through the healing on these pages. I hope that when you forget, these pages will help you remember how to be.

Welcome, beloved, to a journey of healing, in time.

IN MIND, BODY, HEART, & SPIRIT |

body rites is a holistic healing journey. I want to explain what that means, as a foundation for your experience, and also as a potential way of healing in life. Oftentimes, when we think about mental and emotional health, we center fitness of the mind. This is important, and also it inherently comes with limitations. Focusing on the mind as a singular means of healing is rooted in the beginnings of the field of psychology in the Western world, created by white men within systems that serve white people and oppress all others. The tools that were innovated in the psychology field's beginnings and beyond were used to establish superiority by way of biased and defective "science and proof" that others, namely folks of African ancestry were inferior. Consequently, this has influenced how we understand and relate to our mental health as individuals and in community as Black beings.

We have adopted westernized beliefs/value systems that have shaped our lives and our healing is no exception. I use the word "adopted" loosely. What feels more true is that Black beings have been conditioned under the institution of colonization. Our minds, bodies, and our healing have been manipulated through enslavement and its contemporary descendants and manifestations. This is an intrusive, abrasive, and abusive process that continues to impact how we move in the world, how we understand it, how we relate to ourselves/others, how we shrink/stand in our power, how we are disjointed from our personal truth, and how we externalize our trust in determining what is best for us on our healing journeys. And for multi-generations we have practiced forgetting as a means of survival.

> *when you turn the last page,*
> *I pray your arms are joyously tired from*
> *holding all that you remembered and discovered.*

While many of us can recognize the overt ways in which historical oppression colors our present experiences, some of us may have a harder time sensing into the insidious nature of colonization and the harm it causes. The enslavement of African people and colonization forbade our people's use of their indigenous medicines, access to sacred plants and herbs, music, language, movement, foods, and spiritual tools. We were people deeply connected to the elements—earth, water, air, and fire. We held our elders close and our ancestors in sacred embrace. We experienced elevation and healing as a collective, in community.

body rites, as a holistic healing journey, anchors into the practice of decolonizing our medicine and reclaiming our body sovereignty. It reaches back into our indigenous roots and land-based healing. It centers remembering as a means of survival. We are not just minds or brains. We are not simple, compartmentalized beings. We are complex, whole, dynamic beings and all of our aspects/parts are interconnected. Thus, attending to our healing is not merely a mental exercise. When we are grounded in these truths—remembering and decolonizing our medicine—our healing can take on a different path. In this context, the practice of decolonizing is to untangle and unbraid ourselves and ways of being from oppressive conditioning. It is to reach back into the wells of wisdom and traditions that we once knew, those that were lost in surviving global colonization so that healing is shaped from the inside, rather than controlled from the outside. Ultimately, it is hoped that this unbraiding process will incite memory of body sovereignty—the knowing that your body is yours.

Some notes on decolonizing healing |

Unlearning is a long haul, but I have one tip to root the decolonization of your healing practices.

QUESTION EVERYTHING. Many of us are already doing this work; some of us may be afraid to ask questions because we fear the answers will challenge everything we have come to believe or have been taught. It might. There is no shame in that.

> *The practice of fear is oppression working.*
> *Fear is oppression spreading out inside.*
> *It is the embodiment of colonization.*

So, here's a list of questions to keep close and space to add your own, in the spirit of remembrance and accountability. I invite you to ask yourself:

- Are the values I practice also tools that have been used to oppress me and my communities?
- Where did it come from—that belief, value, energy, judgment? Where did I learn this?
- Where did the fear come from? Is it mine or was it left with me? If it was left with me, was it to protect me or to protect them/others/oppressors?
- Why am I afraid of remembering what has been forgotten?
- Do my values and practices dilute my authenticity and truth?

body rites

OK, so how do we put this all into practice in healing from sexual trauma? I see you asking questions. I invite you to consider shifting your healing orientation into a paradigm that inspires your remembrance—one that assists you in the whole beautifully complex being that you are. Even as you are reading this, I invite you to notice how it feels to be affirmed in your wholeness in this exact moment. *body rites* is grounded in a **mind–body–heart–spirit** orientation that I discovered in my own healing journey and in holding sacred therapeutic space for others. I have witnessed its power and reach and am honored to share it with you. At the base of this paradigm of healing, is an understanding of T R A U M A. Trauma affects the whole being (more on this in the next chapter), and thus, healing can be profound when it holds the whole being as well—mind, body, heart, spirit. The mind aspect is concerned with our beliefs, truths/untruths, how we think about ourselves and the world. The body, perhaps one of the most neglected aspects in the mental health field, is about how our lived experiences manifest physically, physiologically, and energetically. The heart part regards our relationships and love for self and others. Lastly, the spirit facet is about our relationships with a god or a higher power/self, sense of purpose, intuition, and our ancestors.

IN FLOW—A WORD ON HOW |

body rites is the first of its kind—an embodied healing journey and holistic resource/workbook of rituals for Black women, femmes, and nonbinary survivors of sexual assault. This workbook is a gentle guide and liaison, exploring the impact of sexual trauma on the mind, body, heart, and spirit. It is an invitation to heal holistically, drawing upon indigenous medicine, psychophysiology, lived body wisdom, trauma-informed embodiment practices, and kinship/ancestral connections.

Most urgently, it is a series of intimate conversations with your self and remembrance that healing lives at the core of your intuition. Additionally, because it is time that we reclaim our voices in shaping healing spaces, I have also written a brief epilogue for helping professionals that journey with and hold space for our communities.

All this in mind, there is no wrong way to do this. I suppose that if there is a right way, it would be something only you could determine. I know that beginning a new healing venture can be overwhelming though, so I would like to offer some suggestions for using the workbook. Please know that you are supported in discerning your method and your path through.

Disclaimers & Invitations

I believe that we have much of what we need inside to heal. I believe that because many of us have forgotten, in order to survive, that we might have to reach back or more deeply to retrieve the wisdom that exists within us and just beyond us. To this end, I anticipate that in these pages you will remember things you have forgotten, things that you did not realize you knew, and things that you need for this exact time. And if your heart is open to it, I think you might discover some new things too.

This workbook has been written with the utmost thoughtfulness and intentionality. It has been designed to be experienced in the order it is presented, but I know healing ain't linear! The earlier sections are written to support your settling in, gathering tools for what's to come, and to ground in context. The middle sections guide you through the work and embodied healing practices, collecting and deepening rituals along the way. At last, we close in the clutch of our ancestors and liberatory self-reflection. However, if you find yourself drawn to explore sections spontaneously, please do with all your fervor. Know that you do not need permission or instructions for your journey. The journey is yours.

You will also notice that the workbook is beautifully decorated from beginning to end. I believe that aesthetics hold our gaze steady so that we can see more. They help us to be present, and they remind us of the beauty within and around us. I encourage you to invite the aesthetics into your experience; to notice what they invoke; and to observe when they reflect, hold, or stir you. Each piece of art on these pages has been meditatively created in collaboration with one of my favorite beings on the planet, dr. shyma el sayed. In many moments throughout, you will be invited to witness, create, engage with, and write on the art. Be free in your expressions and in this space that is all yours—I hope you will write, draw, paint, imagine, collage, or tea or coffee stain all over it.

Behold, beloved, be moved by your healing art.

OVERVIEW OF TRAUMA-INFORMED CARE HISTORY, WHY, & PRINCIPLES |

There are many roots anchoring this journey. Years of study, living, healing, experimenting, channeling, being, unlearning, and unfolding. There are the medicinal contributions of elders and my revered teachers. There is the rich soil of empty space on these pages that awaits planting of your healing intentions. There is the fundamental truth that you deserve healing space that understands the power of personal choice, that celebrates you being in control of you and your body, and that is trauma informed.

Trauma informed, trauma sensitive, trauma conscious, and other varied expressions speak to this fundamental value system. While trauma-informed care has become quite the trend and buzz of the well-being world, many are relating to it as a principle when it is a culture (shift). I am sharing this with you for two reasons. One, because I also value transparency and want you to know what I know to bolster healthy vigilance on your healing journey, here and beyond. Two, I want you to know that you deserve this kind of care in every area of your life. So, let's get into it!

I love discovering synergy and collective consciousness. This is what it felt like when I stumbled on the trauma-sensitive ideology in 2011. I was in graduate school at the time, constantly navigating competing energies between my intuition and the "science" of the field of psychology. As a novice clinician, I was being taught to ground my orientation/approach to therapy in evidence-based practices, or practices that were deemed legitimate and effective through rigorous research and clinical trials. Many of these research studies excluded or underrepresented the communities I work with and come from. It often felt like an act of betrayal to anchor my clinical orientation in theories written by white folks who were studying the lived experiences of white folks. Additionally, I felt immense discomfort with the inherent power dynamic connected to these theories, particularly in ways that seemed to disempower the clients/communities I was working with. Enduring individual and systemic violations that abate personal/collective power and choice is difficult enough, but to then ask folks to entrust their care to spaces that maintain those same values was painfully counterintuitive for me.

I had begun experimenting with centering intuition, self-determination, spontaneous insight, and the body narrative as medicinal and a covert theoretical orientation, when I discovered trauma-sensitive pedagogy. To be clear, trauma sensitive, interchangeably known as trauma informed or trauma conscious, is not a psychological theory. It is a way of being and holding and, in my opinion, a non-negotiable practice. While I will not be offering a comprehensive overview of trauma-informed care here, I want to highlight some of the most essential themes.

Trauma-informed care, as a framework, is rooted in anti-oppression and anti-racism efforts. It intimately knows that the healing journey is complex, nuanced, person-specific, and that it is one of bottomless choices. It is an accountability practice for professionals that hold space for healing and, more expansively, a culture that we all have a role in shaping and are worthy of. Trauma-informed care prioritizes the lived experiences of survivors, their intersectional identities, multiplicitous contexts, and with regard to our beloved Black humanity, the impact of targeted harm across generations. In this same vein, to be trauma informed is to know vulnerability in healing and to avoid causing further harm and/or retraumatization as much as possible. Most imminently, trauma-informed care celebrates and nourishes the truth that every being everywhere is their own guru or awo.

I have condensed and presented the primary trauma-informed care tenets below. I invite you to notice what feels resonant and keep them close as you journey forward here and also in the world. May they become the bare minimum standard for you and all of us in healing. The National Sexual Violence Resource Center (2011) identifies the following core principles of trauma-informed care as safety, trust, choice, collaboration, empowerment, and cultural competence. I have modified collaboration as cocreation and added consciousness and self-determination as additional principles in my practice, in efforts to fill in gaps. Each of the workbook sections to follow stand on these trauma-informed care principles as part of the foundation for healing. Below, I have created a quick reference and affirmation guide of trauma-informed care principles to return to as needed. You're invited to add and/or edit the affirmations as it feels right.

It is my deep belief that self-determination in the healing process (and in general!) is transformative, urgent, and a powerful path to sustainable freedom. While this is not explicitly named as a principle in the trauma-informed care tutelage, I am naming it here as vital and worshipped in this healing space. I hope that you feel that throughout.

safety | to feel safe in your being, in relationship, in healing space, and in the world is your birthright. It is a process and takes time. People and places can intend to inspire feelings of safety, but only you can determine your experience of safety.

{Affirmation} Feeling safe takes time.

trust | is earned and grows in relationship. It lives in the heart space and can change based on experience.

{Affirmation} I know when trust is here because I feel it in my heart.

choice | making choices on the healing journey is an act of power and reclamation. In the practice of making choices, survivors are able to reconnect with their intuition and become an active informant to their care. Receiving invitations to choose between options, to choose timing, and to opt in/out are all examples of what this can look like.

{Affirmation} Making choices in healing is an act of power and something to be reclaimed.

cocreation | is a dance. It requires mutual respect and sees a survivor as a decision maker and part of a team.

{Affirmation} My voice is important in shaping the care I receive.

empowerment | happens when others inherently believe that a survivor's voice, sense of power, and knowing matter. Empowerment looks like believing what a survivor is saying about their experience and needs, centering their personal strengths in their care, and bolstering their confidence along the way.

{Affirmation} I am worthy of having a support team that believes me and celebrates my strengths.

cultural competence | is one aspect of offering competent care. At minimum, all professionals on a survivor's team should be competent in their skillset and operate within their respective scopes of practice. This includes knowing their limitations, biases, and blind spots when working with marginalized identities and the potential impact of causing harm. Helpers should center the lived experience of survivors and their identity intersections when making recommendations.

{Affirmation} My story is rich and complex in its layers, and I deserve care that can competently and responsibly hold space for me.

self-determination | allows a survivor to decide who and how they want to BE. In the healing space, it supports intuitive and informed decision making that feels aligned with what is needed in the moment even when it departs from what others think is best for them.

{Affirmation} self-determination is a path to freedom.

Freedom + choice + intuition
"These are things that were lost. These are the things you will take back.
They belong to you."

The journey is yours

I invite you to take a moment to remember how you discovered this book, to allow yourself to travel back in time. How did it happen? Was it a gift from a loved one? A social media post? Were you browsing the shelves of your favorite book store? What feelings came up? What made you light up? What made it feel right, and like the right time? I invite you to take a few breaths into these acknowledgements. Openings for healing can be so serendipitous, curious, so mysterious even. Do you trust your drawing to this journey? I do. The moment this book landed in your hands, is when the ceremony began. As we move forward, I want to encourage some reliable practices that you can return to throughout. I invite you to think about this as an opening ritual.

"Triggers are visits from the past."
—Bea Hyacinthe of Love & Kindness Wellness

TRIGGER + CONTENT/CARE WARNING |

I encourage you to continue checking in with yourself about your capacity as you progress through the workbook. This work is personal and for many can excavate painful memories—our own and those we are connected to. When you notice that your body is asking for a break or distance from the material, I invite you to pause, use the tools you'll be accumulating throughout, or opt out perhaps returning to triggering sections later, if that feels right. Oftentimes, when folks are triggered, they are encouraged to ground, find stillness, and recenter in the present moment. These can be great options. However, I encourage you to experiment with *moving through* the trigger—exploring movement as an alternative to stillness—this might look like rocking, swaying, stomping, stretching, or a gentle flow of shapes. This helps the body to move through the traumatic memory, as opposed to tucking it away or creating the climate for it to get lodged somewhere inside. When we move through it, we free up space in our bodies. You get to decide what feels right in those moments. Know that you can take your time and choose the pace.

Sweet code of healing

To begin, I would like to offer some suggestions for agreements you might make with yourself and invite you to write in your own. These agreements, or sweet code of healing as I affectionately call them, are gentle intentions and ways to hold yourself in compassion and accountability. As you edit these and add your own, you might consider what you need from yourself to promote ease, what you need when things get hard, what helps you to follow through, and what gets in the way.

- Set some healing intentions; what would you like to happen in this journey?
- Be honest with yourself.
- Listen to and honor your body/intuition. Everything is an option.
- Know that your choices are supported.
- Modify, tweak, and adjust as you need, as much as you need.
- Hold yourself gently and with love.
- Get your support squad together (up next!)
- Ask for support when you need it.
- Use your self-care plan generously (more on this in a bit!)
- Determine your own pace. This will help you to see the journey through.
- Do your best.
- _____
- _____
- _____

body rites

Support squad

Dear beloved, having quality and dependable support is essential! I encourage you to consider what this means for you. Who are the people, where are the places, and what are the things that encourage feelings of safety, being held, and nonjudgment perhaps. This list might include therapists, friends, family, pets, partners, elders, or spiritual advisors. If it feels OK, I invite you to selectively tell them you are embarking on this journey and how you'd like them to support you. You may even feel inspired to invite close friend–survivors to grab their own copy and journey through the workbook with you.

Who are your people?

How do you like/need to be supported?

What are the barriers to asking for what you need?

How would you like to share your support needs with your people?

Self-care plan

We have begun the conversation (and the work!) of decolonizing our healing. I might argue that self-care is at the center of that. When we can see ourselves at the center of our concentric circles, with passionate conviction, our healing flourishes. This is indeed a paradigm shift for Black women. We have been conditioned and nonconsensually obligated to the CARETAK-ING of others, at the expense of ourselves. We have internalized an ethos and value system that disturbingly affirms selflessness as aspirational, self-care as selfish, and self-abandonment as a determination of worth. To be clear beloved, I am not coming for you. *I am you.* This mayhem did not miss me. I want to instigate your critical side eye and inspire a new way of being in time. As we know, healing doesn't happen overnight, but an inner rebellion can commence at any time.

I invite you to rebel, beloved, perhaps by crafting a self-care plan that you can relentlessly return to throughout this ceremony. First, by considering your relationship with self-care as it is at present, by reimagining it with you at the center, and lastly identifying barriers to following through. I'll walk with you through it. Bear in mind that this is JUST the beginning, a foundation. Your self-care game will undoubtedly change and evolve in these ceremonial pages.

You're invited to offer yourself time to reflect on the journaling prompts on the following page.

JOURNALING PROMPTS |

- What were your earliest examples of self-care?
  - How did you observe your caretakers caring for themselves?
  - How did they manage stress?
  - How do you think culture and gender play a role?
- What's your current self-care situation?
  - What are your favorite self-care activities?
  - How often do you do something just for you?
  - Do you feel like you are most often pouring from a full or empty cup?
- What are the barriers that get in the way of you doing you?
  - physical
  - emotional
  - logistical
- You're invited to take up the space below and on the following journaling page to reimagine self-care |
  - Things you might say to your loved ones when you need time for yourself:
    - e.g., I am feeling _____ and could really use _____
    - _____
    - _____
    - _____
- Ways you can take care of yourself. You're invited to include self-care activities that are already in your practice as well as those you'd like to reconnect with in each of the following areas.
  - Mind
  - Body
  - Heart
  - Spirit

body rites

COLLECTED WOUNDS & HISTORY OF SEXUAL ASSAULT OF BLACK WOMEN & THEIR BODIES |

These pages are coated with the wisdom of my ancestors and years of my personal and academic study. Can I share a story with you about this? I was living in Chicago, while in graduate school, when I truly leaned into a practice of noticing. There were a few things going on during this time that I attribute to the deepening awareness of spirit and intergenerational and ancestral traumas as a real thing. I was in a new place, far removed from everything I had ever known. It was a fresh slate with blank neutral space for me to engage all of my senses without interference from some of the familiar noise. I had an intimate and consistent yoga practice, which was a tumultuous freedom journey into presence and embodiment. I learned quickly, when I am present and IN my body, I am more sensitive to the layered experience of sensation, discomfort, pain, story, energy, and spiritual consciousness. I began noticing all the manifestations of these layers in my body, just beyond my being, in my interactions with others, and in the environments I occupied. The third occurrence that stood out was my relationship with writing. I describe myself as a deep feeler, and as a child, someone that could intuit and sense into things I did not yet have the life experience to understand. When I was writing my doctoral dissertation, the conception of some of what I will be sharing with you, I would write pages and pages only to return to them and not recognize what had been written. It occurred to me that I was channeling, my writing a conduit for my/our ancestor-survivors to share their voices, stories, and healing wisdom. And here we are, again.

I give thanks for our ancestors.
Whose healing outlasts their lifespans.
Whose wounds bring wisdom
And whose children stand in truth and power
In spite of . . .

Sexual assault is any type of sexual contact or behavior that occurs without consent. Falling under the definition of sexual assault are sexual activities including but not limited to forced sexual intercourse, forcible sodomy, molestation, incest, fondling, and attempted rape (Tjaden & Thoennes, 2000) and most recently recognized, stealthing. Experiences of sexual abuse/assault can happen at any age/any point in the life span; they can occur once or habitually, and be perpetuated by a stranger or more commonly someone known to the person.

Sexual assault in colonial America

Understanding the historical context of sexual assault, including American culture as the sexual exploiter of enslaved Africans for centuries, is vital to realizing the complexity of surviving the trauma as Black women and beings. Enslavement of Africans was an attempt to suppress their sexual nature that was deemed animalistic by those in power (Collins, 2000; Roberts, 1998; Wyatt, 1992). Enslaved African women were often arbitrarily assigned a sexual partner and ordered to mate, used as rewards for enslaved men after a day's work, were at the beck and call of their enslaver's sexual demands, and generally used for sexual recreation (Brownmiller, 1975). Post emancipation, sexual assault and rape were used as political weapons and terror tactics (Hall, 1983; Roberts, 1998). Being free did not by any means guarantee that a Black woman would not be sexually assaulted. The misconception that Black women could not be raped due to conditioned beliefs that they were sexually promiscuous and inferior have been imprinted on the cultural heritage of America and have contributed to common myths of sexual assault, objectification of Black women, the sexual politics around Black womanhood, strain of help seeking/reporting, and a wounded culture of silence (Brownmiller, 1975; Collins, 2000).

Sexual assault in the 21st century

Sexual assault is arguably one of the most destructive crimes against a person—against humanity. While there have been decades of movements dedicated to ending cycles of sexual violence against women in particular, the prevalence of sexual assault seems to perpetually defy them. A quick investigation into the prevalence of sexual assault is staggering. According to the National Intimate Partner and Sexual Violence Survey (2015), one in five women in the United States experienced completed or attempted rape during their lifetime. One in four Black girls will be sexually abused before the age of 18, and one in five Black women are survivors of rape (The National Center on Violence Against Women in the Black Community, 2018). Research has also shown that Black girls and women 12 years and older experience higher rates of sexual assault and rape than white, Asian, and Latina girls (Planty et al., 2013). Transgender and nonbinary individuals are victimized at higher rates, with almost half (47%) reporting being sexually assaulted at some time in their lives (U.S. Transgender Survey, 2015). The more layered and intersecting the identities, the higher the numbers go. And naturally given systemically rooted ruptures between Black communities and law enforcement agencies and the taboo of discussing sexual abuse, the numbers are limited, and likely severely lower than actual accounts of sexual assault. "For every 15 Black women who are raped, only one reports her assault" (Hart & Rennison, 2003).

The stories live on in our bodies—our own, our communities, and our ancestors. They spread out inside us and take up space. They fester and create dis-ease. They ache and scrape our insides in hearing resonant stories that belong to others. This is a reality so many of us have been living with for generations. A reality that we can change our relationship with, by holding space for ourselves, mind, body, heart, and spirit.

body rites

As you are reading, you may be noticing some things in your own being. Perhaps sensations of resistance or maybe those of recognition/being seen. I invite you, beloved, to be with it, embracing it as an important part of this journey. You might offer yourself a cleansing breath, inhaling from the crown of your head and exhaling a white light cascade of breath over the body and down into the earth. Take your time.

There is more to discover here, in the acknowledgements of our collected and collective wounds. These are the myriad displays of our ancestors' and our elder family members' stories living on in our bodies, our patterns, and family dynamics. We know things that we ourselves do not have the lived experiences for, and we carry with us in our bodies their wounds. It is my honor to guide you in the sacred revelation of this light and dark throughout our ceremony. We will take special care to explore these connections in upcoming sections.

LIBATION RITUAL FOR ANCESTRAL SUPPORT |

In African spiritual traditions, commencement of community gathering—in celebration, seasonal change, or ceremony—includes honoring of the ancestors. This acknowledgement can take the form of libation, prayer, song, dance, or ritual to name a few of many options. That said, it feels just right to invite our ancestors into ceremonial support for you, for them, for all of us. It gives me indulgent chills to imagine that each time this ritual is offered, that more elevated ancestors come forward in support of your healing and the collective.

All you need for the libation ritual is a live plant and a glass of water. Remember! There will be numerous times to begin with this ritual and to make it your own in the pages to come if you choose. You can also make this offering directly to the earth if you prefer or if a plant is not available.

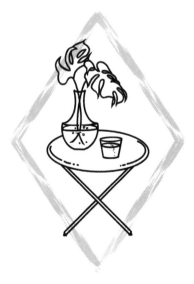

Instructions for libation ritual

As you're ready, hold your glass of water to your chest if you are able. Notice its coolness as you begin to invite cool breath into the body, feeling it pass through the nostrils on the inhale and exhaling sending that breath into the glass for about three rounds of breath. You're invited to begin recalling the names of your most beloved ancestors—those you think most fondly of, who inspire you, or those you feel close to. These can be relatives from your own bloodline or those you have never met but want to reverence and draw support from in your healing journey. When it feels right, begin saying each of those ancestors' names out loud, pouring a splash of water into the plant or earth as you simultaneously speak each of their names. An offering of water poured into the earth or plant honors their lives and sacred legacies and invites peaceful relationship. You're encouraged to stay here until it feels complete. Notice any sensations or emotions that arise as you observe yourself, your body, and the air around you.

Weep.
Tears are embodied libations.
Let salted water fall out of you.
Into your hands.
Rub them together.
Generate heat between them, create fire.
Feel their blood.
The rich rivers of our ancestors flowing inside you.
This is ritual and an opening.

body rites

body rites

1st Journey | *settling IN*

AN INVITATION—EMBODIMENT |

This is an INvitation, beloved . . . a reaching out, to call you back inside and into your bodies. Living IN Black bodies ain't easy. We have been enduring and trying to feel safe in bodies with targets on them for generations. This keeps us suspended in fight, flight, freeze, submit, and tend and befriend modes. We have been INternalizing, hiding, and dismissing our emotions and experiences. That turns INto dis-ease. We carry the stories of our ancestors with us in our cells, our blood, and body memory. We survive being violated and assaulted in these bodies, having the stories imprinted on our senses and energy body. This can feel like living in a crime scene.

Embodiment is a birthright.
It is to come into this world spirited and present with our selves.
It is to practice presence in the body, it is to BE in the body.
To know it. To sense it. To believe it.

This journey, *settling IN*, the first of four, supports your easing into the *body rites*, exploring the lived-body experience, recalibrating to holistic/body-centered healing ideology, and understanding the impact of sexual trauma on the brain and nervous systems. And we begin the practice of embodiment through exploration of grounding tools, attunement to the body through self-reflection, and through creation of opening and closing rituals.

The opening

I am calling you IN beloved, into ceremony and intimate pursuit of residing within. For some of us, we may be returning to a place we once knew and fully claimed. Expansive and vibrant presence in the body. For others, it may feel like a journey into a birthright-place that is both unknown and longed for. I invite you to (re)imagine what it looks, feels, and tastes like to fully live in your physical body. What happens when you allow curiosity to be one of your journey companions? You might notice that the edges of limitation seem to dissolve and the horizon of possibilities beams. When you're ready, you might continue your exploration and imagining through a gentle meditation and scan of your body with curiosity.

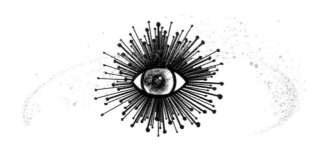

As it feels right, I invite you to choose a comfortable physical shape. You might choose a seated shape, one lying down, or even standing if it feels right. If you're able, you're invited to choose a shape that allows some part of your body to touch the floor/earth. Know that you are supported in choosing what feels right for your body in every moment. Once you've settled on a shape |

- You might begin focusing on the part of your body meeting the earth, allowing yourself to grow from that place in all directions, into the earth, south, north, east, and west of you.

- Maybe the eyes want to make a choice to close, gaze down, or remain open.

- Briefly observe the breath and make any adjustments that feel supportive, perhaps slowing it down, expanding it, or asking it to begin and end in the tummy.

- Imagine that you are able to trace the outline of your body with your mind. You might be reminded of a school-aged activity, where you traced your hand or a classmate's body with a crayon. With that same sweetness and curiosity, continue slowly tracing your body's edges in your mind's eye.

- You might observe with your inner awareness the shape you created.

- When it feels right, return your focus to the breath. On the inhales feel yourself filling up your shape to its edges, and settle INto yourself on the exhales. If it feels OK, you might linger here for 10–15 breaths.

- You might take a moment to notice something that changed, feels different, or better than when you began meditating.

- Guide yourself back into the present and take a few moments to reflect on the following journaling page if you'd like.

body rites

Trauma is a subjective and whole being experience, violating mind, body, heart, and spirit. Our modern society is only beginning to recognize this fundamental truth. When I was in graduate school, I found myself particularly intrigued with the impact of trauma on the body. Certainly, this was inspired by my own experiences of trauma and my intuitive preference to pursue healing in my body. Years have since passed, and there has been an uptick in acknowledging the lived-body experience, the somatic imprint of trauma, and the innumerable manifestations of sexual trauma on the physical body. It happens to the body.

I mentioned earlier that in the aftermath of sexual trauma it can feel like living in a crime scene. This is one remarkable distinction between other traumatic experiences and sexual trauma. The abuse happens to the body that we live in. We can't pack up and move away. It doesn't become a memory of something hard that happened in a place we once resided. *The body is the place.* I know I don't need to convince you. I know that you know what it's like to BE and live in a body that someone else tried to own. It happens to the body.

Somehow though, the body gets left out of healing spaces. We focus on the mind and tell ourselves that if only we could forget, forgive, deny, think differently about it, and talk through it that we can heal it. For many of us, it may seem counterintuitive and even frightening to center our bodies in healing from sexual trauma. Especially if your body is a place you have been trying to escape, if you feel betrayed by it, or if it seems to provoke unwanted desire/attention. It's not your body's fault.

You deserve to be at home in your body. To take up all the space inside of it. To feel softness at its edges and peace in your blood. To change in it. To be held by it. To share pleasure with it. To rest in it. To make love with it. *These are your body's rites, beloved.*

I believe the body is the medicine. That centering it in the healing journey and searching for its voice can profoundly shift the way we live. May it be so.

> *"The body has a way of calling things forward."*
> —Isabel Adon, Indigenous focusing-oriented therapist

If your body could talk, what would it say? You're encouraged to write and create freely below.

How has trauma changed the way your body feels and functions?

You're invited to take some time to observe and reflect on your lived-body experience. Take a moment to review the INventory below tracking what you sense as true using the following symbols.

- an **O** to indicate resonance with the description. In marking an "O" you are noting that this is an experience you have at present, recently, most often, or chronically.
- a **P** to indicate resonance with the description as something that you have experienced in the past.

***please note this inventory is not intended to be used as a diagnostic tool or indicator of a medical/mental health condition.

__ Flashbacks/reexperiencing traumatic event(s)
__ Feeling easily startled
__ Change in mood
__ Panic attacks
__ Irritability
__ Feeling out of sorts
__ Memory challenges
__ Nightmares
__ Insomnia or trouble sleeping
__ Restlessness
__ Problems focusing/concentrating
__ Change in appetite
__ Body aches/muscle soreness
__ Headaches or migraines
__ Chest tightness/pain

__ Hypertension

__ Rapid heart rate

__ Excessive sweating

__ Significant weight gain/loss

__ Stomach aches/abdominal pain

__ Gastrointestinal issues (e.g., IBS)

__ Acid reflux/indigestion

__ Unexplained changes in menstruation

__ Pain during sex

__ Uterine fibroids

__ Endometriosis

__ Recurrent UTIs

__ Sensitive bladder

__ Nausea

__ Fatigue

__ Loss or decrease in sexual interest

__ Lump in the throat sensation

__ Feelings of choking

__ Cold limbs or extremities

__ Loss of energy

__ Fainting

__ Feelings of worthlessness

__ Trembling or shaking

__ Shortness of breath

__ Excess energy

__ Dizziness

__ Numbness/tingling in the body

You're invited to take some time with the following diagram making note of places you experience pain, soreness, numbness, discomfort, or disconnection in your body.

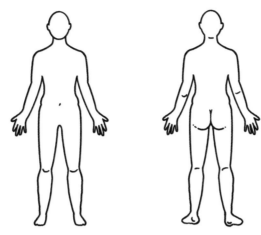

You're encouraged to pause and take a few breaths, noticing all there is in the moment—the discovery, the connections being made, the questions arising, and the confirmation. It happens to the body. And the body remembers. It tucks the sensations, energy, and painful memories into its tissues, organs, and muscles; pours the shock into its blood; fossilizes the violation; and screams through aches and pains. The body is loud. You are not making this up.

Take a moment, beloved. Touch three things in your physical space, if it feels right. A furry pillow, a warm salt lamp, a cool table/desk. You are only several pages in and already you are listening to your body. Physical health distress that survivors of sexual violence experience throughout their recoveries are real health problems and are extremely common (Campbell et al., 2003, p. 91). These health issues can be categorized as chronic diseases, non-chronic illnesses, and recurring health problems including but not limited to gastrointestinal symptoms, muscular/skeletal problems, cardiopulmonary symptoms, neurological symptoms, and gynecological issues. Additionally, I'd like to name the negative impact of sexual violence on the energy body as well. My intentions are not to alarm you, rather to assist in illuminating the monumental impact of sexual violation on the body and to invite you into the opportunity to listen to it as a way forward. Of course, you are supported in sharing your insights with your care team (therapists, physicians, healing practitioners) to monitor/assess any serious medical conditions, to inform treatment options, and to make meaning.

You're invited to continue exploring and journaling in the space to follow. As you reflect on what came up, you might also consider when these experiences, sensations, symptoms, or challenges began (e.g., before or after the trauma).

body rites

Brain things

Can we take a lil trip back to middle school biology, beloved? It really does get this deep. Deep in the body, more specifically the brain. Discussions of trauma easily lend to the psychological impact, how our lived experiences affect our minds, imaginations, and hide away in our unconscious. In recent years, conversations about the somatic disruption of trauma emphasize the physiological experience. Bessel van der Kolk, author of *The Body Keeps the Score* (2014), says:

> After trauma the world is experienced with a different nervous system. The survivor's energy now becomes focused on suppressing inner chaos at the expense of spontaneous involvement in their life. These attempts to maintain control over unbearable physiological reactions can result in a whole range of physical symptoms . . . (p. 53)

Just because we can't see it or aren't actively talking about it doesn't mean it is not in-process on the inside. Trauma shocks and is stored in multiple areas of the brain as it relates to the experience itself, memories, and sensations. There are a few parts of the brain touched by trauma I'd like to highlight for extra credit.

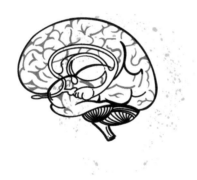

Limbic system | is our primitive or emotional brain that perceives and reacts to threat. Babette Rothschild, author of *The Body Remembers* (2000), describes it as "survival central" in preparing the body for defensive action.

Amygdala | An almond shaped area of the brain that acts as the body's alarm system and emotional memory center, activating fight or flight responses and coactivating freeze, submit, tend, and befriend responses. When the amygdala gets stuck in protective mode, it constantly identifies danger when no immediate threat of danger is present.

Hippocampus | is responsible for abilities to retrieve and store memory, understand concepts, adopt new skills, and links new information to past experiences. In this way, it has an intimate relationship with the amygdala. The hippocampus' intimate relationship with emotional experience, memory, and trauma offers some explanation as to why some survivors are not able to recall cognitive memory/vivid details of what happened to them. To take it further, some survivors have no recollection of their sexual trauma at all. But there's a part(s) that somehow knows, tucked deep inside that may show up as feelings in the body, dreams, aversions, and intense and seemingly random emotional reactions around certain family members. You have a special place in my heart. I believe you. I believe your body.

Thalamus | a relay station that collects sensations from the ears, eyes, and skin and integrates them into autobiographical memory (van der Kolk, 2014, p. 70). "A breakdown of the thalamus explains why trauma is primarily remembered not as a story, a narrative with a beginning, middle, and end, but as isolated sensory imprints: images, sounds, and physical sensations that are accompanied by intense emotions" (p. 70, footnote 17).

Hypothalamus and HPA axis | is our central stress response system. When the amygdala sounds the alarm in response to a threat, it signals the hypothalamus, taps the stress hormone system (e.g., cortisol) and "orchestrates a whole-body response" (van der Kolk, 2014, p. 60).

Speech center | During traumatic stress, the speech center shuts down. This is one reason why many people cannot completely put what happened to them into words, or why in the moment of abuse they were not able to use their voice.

Frontal cortex | When a significant threat presents itself, this part of the brain shuts down to allow instinctive, survival-oriented responses. Thus, higher order thinking, processing, and organizing are offline making it especially challenging or impossible to make complicated decisions, be objective, or accurately interpret the climate of threat.

Somatic nervous system (SomNS) | is "responsible for voluntary movement executed through the contraction of skeletal muscles" (Rothschild, p. 50). This part of the nervous system is often left out of discourse about the impact of trauma on the nervous system. Understanding its function can support understanding the mechanisms by which traumatic events can be remembered implicitly through body posture and movement, despite not having cognitive memories. The body knows, the body remembers.

Beloved, your body has been doing what it needs to survive.
It deserves to be revered for that, not shamed.

Turn up |

When we/our bodies have a subjective experience of feeling threatened or unsafe, our sympathetic nervous system (SNS) is activated. This part of our autonomic nervous system functions involuntarily, assisting us in mobilizing and preparing the body for action by activating physiological responses to protect and defend ourselves. This is most often accompanied by a cluster of physical sensations, including an increase in heart rate, blood pressure, and breathing rate (van der Kolk, 2014, p. 61). While folks might generally associate the SNS with seeking safety, it's not that simplistic. Particularly when we consider the influence of sociopolitical, cultural, familial, and historical/ancestral contexts, *safe* may feel chronically foreign. What might not be sensed as a threat to one person or group of people or body may feel life threatening for another/other groups. Remember this is an involuntary, automatic, physiological response informed by a person's subjective experience, social conditioning, traumatic history, lived experience of the -isms and oppression (e.g., racism, sexism, homophobia). It may also be an unconscious process. What might initially be a response to a threat or traumatic experience, however, may become a way of being or a way of surviving as the nervous system stalls out in a new, activated norm.

WISDOM NOTES

Experiences of chronic stress and complex trauma signal various alarm bells, triggering the body's interconnected systems to help us mobilize and pursue safety. When a person is constantly enduring stress and trauma, the body and its systems are not able to reset/return to a healthy baseline, causing suspension in an activated SNS, excess stress hormones, and imbalance in the endocrine system. Over time this can suppress the immune system and contribute to physical health concerns or dis-ease. This is an urgent consideration given the consequence of embodied inequality as evident in multigenerational, lifespan, and health disparities in folks of African descent all over the diaspora.

Invitation | how do you know when you are turned up?
what sensations or physical changes do you feel in your body?

body rites

Turn down |

This is the sweet spot. The parasympathetic nervous system (PNS) is responsible for supporting rest, digestion, feelings of calm, and feeling low key. The turn down is associated with relaxation of muscles, a slowing heart rate, and a more natural breathing state. Ideally, after a threat or danger passes, the PNS does the work to bring us back to a healthy calm baseline. Ideally, having a calm and balanced nervous system is something all of us experience. But we don't live in an ideal world. Many of us find ourselves hanging out in an activated sympathetic nervous system response—hyperaroused, perhaps hypervigilant, and holding our breath—or a drowning parasympathetic nervous system frozen and acquiescent. Living in Black bodies with all our intersectional identities often comes with the perception and reality of an abundance of threat and danger. These are manifestations of embodied inequality. As survivors of sexual trauma in particular, a large part of the healing journey is training our bodies to experience the benefits of the PNS, to reclaim our birthright.

Having a calm, healthy nervous system is a
privilege when it should be a birthright.

Invitation | be curious about moments and spaces where you are able to feel calm and breathe with ease. consider healthy activities and relationships that nurture sensations of peace and rest. you're invited to make a turn down list below. know that you can return to this list any time to add new options or guide yourself into restoration.

TRAUMA RESPONSES |

I've been mentioning the physiological trauma responses triggered by the perception of threat. Most of us have likely heard someone say, "I was in fight or flight mode" or "I don't know what happened; I just froze." This is the brain at work trying to keep us safe. When the limbic system is doing its thing, there are a few different mechanisms of protection that are potentially signaled, either helping us to mobilize and take effective action or being overwhelmed and collapsing. Chronic stress, danger, traumatic experiences, or the subjective perception of threat can keep us suspended in these intense exhausting modes. *As you review the following descriptions listed, I invite you to notice what resonates as most familiar to you in moments of crisis, fear, and also in regular life happenings. You are encouraged to journal and/or draw what shows up. You might consider what shapes or positions your body tends toward as you read each description. I call these shapes of trauma.*

Fight | you experience fear.

Without thinking your body moves to strike. You are fighting for your life. For your innocence. Or just because that's what you have come to know in time with trauma as a companion. You experience pain. Out of your mouth spills words that cut. Words that you mean . . . maybe words that you don't mean. Words that bury what you wish you could say but can't, because they have been suffocated by the wounds spreading out in your body. You protect you.

Invitation | when you fight, what are you fighting for?

Flight | your body tells you to run, to escape, to find safety.

You storm out, slamming the doors closed behind you. The moment is too much; you're physically present but have escaped your body to find refuge in the corners of the ceiling, in the crevices of your mind, in the ether. Running has become first nature.

Invitation | how do you run, beloved? what are the situations that lead to running/fleeing?

Freeze | moving in any direction feels impossible.

I've wondered if this is what water feels when it's protecting itself from the elements. From pain, from power and control, from time, from the absence of light. You become the deer in headlights, terrified, panicked, stuck, held hostage by fear.

Invitation | ask your body: what are and the elements that precipitate shutdown, immobility, and challenges in verbalizing your truth and boundaries in everyday life?

Submit | submit is not a yes.

It is a dissolving into oneself, until the danger passes. You hear yourself speaking the language of acquiescence. Setting boundaries feels threatening; you feel they are not worth the risk of loss. You've lied to yourself. You think going along with what everyone else wants/thinks makes you more palatable.

Invitation | consider how submitting shows up in your body. is it a blank stare, is it shrinking, is it trembling, a curved back? how often do you ask yourself, "what do I want or need?"

Tend & befriend | also sometimes referred to as fawn response, describes the manner of caretaking as a means of survival.

The ways in which you might be overly concerned with meeting the needs/desires of others to keep yourself safe, even if it is detrimental to you and your body. Tend and befriend, in my opinion, might be one of the most complex of the protective modes because it is entangled with the impact of trauma on our sense of connection, belonging, and social engagement. Tend and befriend and codependency are homies. I imagine that you might be putting some of this together for yourself, but it is especially nuanced when we ponder intergenerational and ancestral influences. More to explore there in the fourth journey.

Invitation | you're encouraged to consider how this shows up in your personal experience(s) and relationships. what does the tension of caretaking at the expense of yourself feel like in your body? what's your earliest memory of tending and befriending? how does it show up in everyday life?

It is tempting, beloved, even now in this moment of reading about yourself on these pages . . . in seeing the holograph of your stories taking shape, and in remembering previous versions of yourself to feel like running, to feel discouraged, or to experience shock in what you are realizing. I invite you, dear one, to hold yourself with bottomless compassion. You might consider thanking your body for doing what it needed to keep you safe, for protecting you, and preserving you. You might also begin to whisper to it permission to pursue peace.

THE BRAIN HAS A HEART: A WORD ON POLYVAGAL THEORY

"We are wired for connection.
Our nervous systems are social structures that find balance
and stability in relationship with others." —Deb Dana, Anchored

Our innate yearning for connection and our ability to heal in relationships lives in the brain. I mentioned earlier, the impact of trauma on the heart—our relationship to self, others, community, and associated themes of trust and betrayal. We experience these ruptures interpersonally and also in our nervous systems. At the nervous system level, interpersonal trauma can compromise a person's ability to feel safe and at ease in the world. Stephen Porges, a professor of psychiatry, "rediscovered two vagal pathways in the nervous system that regulate the heart and provide a face–heart connection to communicate what is happening inside our bodies to other people" (Dana, p. 5, 2021). More specifically, this speaks to the literal brain–heart–community connection that lives within each of us. The vagus nerve, a bundle of nerves that originates in the brainstem, wanders through the body, touching various organs throughout. This has dire implications. Dr. Porges's work led to the development of Polyvagal Theory that helps us to understand the interdependent layers of our nervous system, including the involuntary ways our bodies function to keep us alive, its built-in surveillance system for discerning between safety and danger, and its inherent nature for coregulation in safe connection with others. You may be able to imagine then the science of an interpersonal trauma, from the polyvagal perspective. That when there is harm or a rupture in our sense of connection, our ability to feel safe . . . to regulate is also challenged. And also, it is in our natural wiring for connection as humans and as descendants of the African diaspora that we can heal.

Window of tolerance

When the body spends so much of its energy working overtime in response to perceptions of threat, our natural brain baselines are dysregulated. It can feel like you are running when you are sitting still or on the contrary, that you are perpetually exhausted. In theory, with healthy, balanced nervous systems we can conserve energy, we can rest easy, and meet the needs of our daily life. Coined by Dan Siegel (2012), this is sometimes referred to as the optimal zone of arousal or window of tolerance in which a person is able to function most effectively. When in our respective window of tolerance, we are ripe to have clarity in the way we think and feel, awareness of boundaries (both ours and others), experience empathy, be present in the here and now, and are open to meaningful engagement with others.

When our baselines are disrupted by trauma, chronic stress, or we get stuck in defensive trauma modes, we may discover that we are living outside of our window of tolerance. When this is the case, a few things can happen.

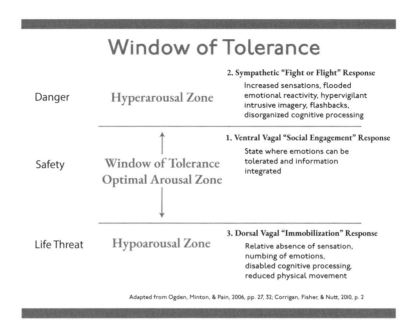

Our window of tolerance shrinks, making it harder to function effectively.

We get bumped up into a hyperarousal zone—which reflects being suspended in activation of fight, flight, and/or freeze defense responses. The hyperarousal zone often presents challenges with states of anxiety, hypervigilance, emotional reactivity/overwhelm, obsessive thoughts, impulsivity, anger, and associated physical sensations (e.g., feeling shaky).

We get bumped down into an underarousal or hypoarousal zone—which occurs when under the pressure of threat, chronic stress, or trauma. The body decompensates and optimal functioning collapses with it. This might look like having little to no energy, feeling disconnected, apathetic, numb, or shutdown with a relative absence of sensation.

Or many of us bounce back and forth between the two. Disharmony in our nervous systems and perpetually living outside your personal window of tolerance can lead to chronic health problems, mental health challenges, ineffective coping, and dissatisfying interpersonal experiences.

You have the power to usher your body into a more harmonious disposition. To reclaim a healthy nervous system; holistically optimize your functioning; experience deeper rest; and nurture a growing sense of safety in your body, emotions, and relationships. These are just several of the possibilities and intentions for our journey together. No(body) is saying it will be easy, and it will likely bring discomfort. Sometimes, in these bodies we inhabit, it can be difficult differentiating between discomfort/unfamiliar and unsafe. As we journey forward and into the unfolding of deep healing, I encourage you to pause and reflect on these two experiences.

Invitation | ask your body if it knows the difference between discomfort/unfamiliar and unsafe. how do you most often navigate discomfort or sensations of unfamiliarity? does this work for you or against you? what do you need from yourself in these instances? how does being unsafe feel different?

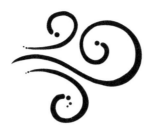

In many healing spaces, folks are expected to disclose their most personal and traumatic stories as a condition or prerequisite to receiving support. Another implicit condition is externalizing our care, decision making, and at worst our intuition to others—healing practitioners/professionals in particular. I sincerely believe that *body rites* is a medicinal and embodied protest to these conditions. I think it is often detrimental to request that a survivor of any trauma relive it in the telling of their stories before they have learned or remembered tools that help them to cope and more importantly to heal. I am affirming that both are available to you here—tools to cope and tools that heal. Perhaps the most potent of the rites in this journey is the repair to intuition. You know what's best for you, beloved. I'm excited for your relentless discovery of this.

Breath as a tool

It is work to BE and breathe through it when everything inside says run.

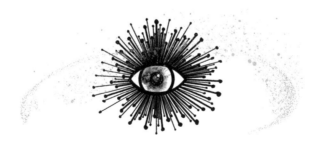

Survivors of trauma often develop shallow breathing patterns consistent with anxiety, hyperarousal, or panic. When overwhelmed, many trauma survivors also tend to unconsciously hold their breath (Emerson & Hopper, 2011, p. 108). Intentional breathwork can be a way to deepen connection with yourself to energize or calm. It can also be used as a focus point when feeling distracted, ungrounded, or flooded with emotions. Attentiveness to your breath as you progress through the workbook will be a great tool to practice and remember. In the upcoming journeys, I'll be sharing a variety of specific breathwork options to add to your toolkit. Here are some breathing tips you might find helpful in the meantime:

- Observe the breath before changing it in any way. Without judgment, choose words, colors, or textures that describe what you are observing.

- Consider what those descriptions or sensations tell you about what could be happening with your breath, your body/nervous system, or life moment (e.g., shallow, cool, deep, strained, coarse, orange, etc.).

- Inhalations are sometimes considered symbolic of our openness to receiving. Short inhalations possibly reflect challenges receiving support or goodness.

- Exhalations, on the other hand, can be evidence of challenges letting go or releasing.

- Holding the breath, my personal favorite, could be a manifestation of bracing or anticipating that something bad is going to happen. You know the old saying, waiting for the other shoe to drop.

- Once you are able to notice HOW you're breathing, you can then make intuitive adjustments to help in the moment. Slowing it down, deepening, expanding, and equalizing are all wonderful options. Spend some time breathing with the adjustments you've made, maybe 10–20 breath cycles if it feels right.

- Be patient, dear one. Our minds are used to wandering all over the place, and many of us certainly aren't accustomed to being present with ourselves and our bodies. You should expect to be distracted or taken off track. It's all good. Ease back in by gently bringing your awareness to caring for your breath.

- Let the thoughts come and go, a catch-n-release. It's possible you might have thoughts like "I can't do this" or "I feel stupid." Try your best not to pull the thread of those thoughts, we all know how that ends up. Instead, you may envision that the inhalations and exhalations are gentle waves washing unhelpful thoughts or distractions away.

- Breathing changes us, literally. Before you shift out of your breathing practice, you might notice what changed and what didn't. Using words, colors, or textures may feel useful here too.

- Practice does not make perfect. Why did they tell us that growing up?! Practicing will not make perfect, but practicing these breathing tools will change you . . . and your body.

Peaceful sacred place | a meditation

In retraining your body to experience peace, it may be helpful to have some quick retreat spaces in mind (pun intended). During times of overwhelm or feeling triggered, retreating to a peaceful sacred space in your mind can be a salve to the nervous system. Further, it is actively choosing to activate the parasympathetic nervous system that supports pacing and tolerance of the sensations that show up in the embodied healing process. Let me nip this in the bud. This is fundamentally different than passively drifting off or dissociation, in that you are choosing to visit a peaceful place in your mind as a healing practice for you and your body; as opposed to involuntarily escaping pain or inner chaos.

When you're ready, I invite you to choose a physical shape or posture for the *peaceful sacred place meditation*. You're encouraged to read through the instructions in full before beginning and returning to journal and draw once you're done.

- You're invited to choose a physical seated shape for your meditation in a quiet space, bringing any pillows or blankets close for extra comfort.
- If it feels OK, you might take a few breaths inhaling through the nose and exhaling out the mouth, imagining that you can release any mental, emotional, or physical distractions.
- Once you're settled in the shape you've chosen, you might allow the eyes to make a choice—closing, softly gazing down, or remaining open.
- Remember the ground is there. See if you can feel its stability under your body or being supported by the furniture you are sitting on.
- Observe the breath and offer any intuitive adjustments that feel supportive—expanding, slowing, elongating.
- When it feels like the right time, you might begin imagining or remembering a peaceful sacred place. Perhaps by focusing on the space between your eyebrows, your inner eye, you might be able to see this place in vivid detail. Notice all there is. Go all out in creating this place that is just yours. Or sink into remembering this place and all the pleasant nostalgia it brings. You're invited to experience this peaceful sacred place with all of your senses.
- What does it look like?
- What sounds are you able to hear?
- What is there to touch?
- Are there any soothing scents?
- What is there to taste?
- How does your heart and body feel in this space?
- It will be tempting to invite others into this peaceful sacred place; however, you are strongly encouraged to protect it as a space that is just for you.
- Once you have been able to visualize your peaceful sacred place, you're encouraged to take 10 to 20 breaths BEING in it.

- When it feels right, take a mental picture and gently guide yourself back into the present. Noticing how you feel the same or different since you began the meditation.

- When you're ready you might blink the eyes open if they are closed, remember the ground is there, and perhaps bring some micro-movements into the body.

If you'd like, you might capture your peaceful sacred place on the page by drawing a picture of it or writing a detailed description. Some questions you might consider reflecting on:

- How were you when you were there?

- What do you notice about how your mind and body feel after the meditation?

- Are there some moments you can think of that may be a good time to visit your peaceful sacred place?

OPENING & CLOSING RITUALS |

This *body rites* ceremony is hella sacred, y'all. You'll be weaving in and out at your own pace. I invite you to imagine what rituals you'd like to practice along the way. Our demanding world has a way of sucking us in and spitting us out; everything blending together with no clear perforation between beginnings and endings. How do you open and close, beloved?

When you picture yourself picking up your *body rites* book for some healing time, how will you begin? How will you transition from what you were doing before and into this special place? How will you ease back in to the other things that need time from you? If it feels right, you might consider designing an opening and closing ritual for yourself below. Keep it simple! We are more likely to follow through with the rituals that bring us ease instead of extra complications.

WISDOM NOTES

Here are a few ritual ideas to get you going.

- Light a candle

- Say a prayer

- Make a cup of tea

- Play a special song or playlist

- Write an affirmation

- Open with the libation ritual or ask elevated ancestors for support

- Smudge your physical space with a sacred smoke

- Place your hands on your heart and take a few breaths

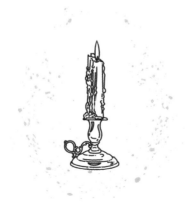

body rites

How do you want to open?

What would be helpful to close and supportive for transitioning back into your day?

2nd Journey | *the work*

This journey deepens *the work*, as a modified and abbreviated version of my 10-week holistic workshop series for survivors, *healing on the mat*. *Healing on the mat* is rooted in Africana Womanist theory and centers the needs and lived experiences of Black women, femmes, and nonbinary survivors. Sibling survivors of the global majority have also found resonance in what it offers. The *healing on the mat* workshop series is grounded in research about the psychophysiological impact of sexual trauma, trauma-informed yoga as an effective treatment option, and centers intentions to heal in mind, body, heart, and spirit. While every survivor has their own special journey and experience, some of the therapeutic benefits of *healing on the mat* are that it helps foster an internal sense of safety, agency, and choice; nurtures capacity for self-awareness and self/coregulation, and provides a way to practice making choices in relationship to one's body.

The body holds so much and often the words we have don't create the opening for the release we might need in the body. Intuitively this makes so much sense, particularly when I reach back into the wisdoms of African spirituality and cultural practices. In many African traditions, movement is the centerpiece of any moment of significance, healing, rite of passage, or community gathering. Further, we have been in conversation about all the ways our lived experiences crystallize or become captive in our bodies. Being a mover myself, dancing since I was a little girl, being a dedicated student of West African dance and a yogi, it was a natural choice to anchor *healing on the mat* in body-centered practices.

One of the hallmarks of *healing on the mat* is trauma-informed yoga. Capturing the history of yoga in its entirety is beyond these pages, however, I'd like to briefly explore the origins and principles as is relevant in healing from sexual trauma. Tracing the history of yoga is a tedious journey in and of itself, as there are varying opinions as to what region of the world from which it emerged. Yoga as it is known in the Western world is most commonly linked to the 5,000-year-old practice of yoga in India in the context of Hinduism (Emerson & Hopper, 2011). Research has also indicated that yoga has African origins and was practiced in Egypt for about 10,0000 years and is known as Kemetic Yoga (Ashby, 2005). You may be able to mentally reference an image of Egyptian gods and goddesses on tomb walls or in hieroglyph artifacts. Although the meaning of yoga is expansive and fluid and eventually may come to mean something subtly different to each of us, the Sanskrit translation of yoga means to yoke or unite. "Many believe that yoga is first and foremost an 'inquiry into being,' an invitation for those curious about what it means to be alive," and an investigation into the subjective experience of being (Emerson & Hopper, 2011, p. 26).

The health benefits of yoga have been well documented as a therapeutic option for reducing the effects of trauma on mental health (Ross & Thomas, 2010; Dick et al., 2014; Yamasaki, 2022, p. 35). *Healing on the mat* heavily leans on trauma-informed yoga as a healing tool. Remember those trauma-informed healing practices and affirmations I shared in the welcome section? I invite you to imagine having a yoga practice grounded in each of those principles. In violations that occur between humans—particularly in sexual trauma—choice, power, and control are stolen. What I love about trauma-informed yoga is that it offers an embodied practice of re-claiming what was lost—power, control, and choice in relationship to the body—"by making small, manageable choices in relation to one's body" (Emerson & Hopper, 2011, p. 45). As my dear friend and colleague says, "it is a supportive inquiry and an invitation for survivors to come into their own bodies, on their own terms" (Yamasaki, 2022). This has been profoundly impactful to my own healing. On the mat, I reclaim, reflect, and make infinite choices and off the mat I put these discoveries to work. It's a beautifully woven parallel to the healing process. I am not alone in this. Witnessing the transformation of survivors in the *healing on the mat* workshop series has been incredibly moving.

Can we talk about the elephant in the room? Some of you might be thinking, "yoga is for thin white people." I know how it is. When you don't see people that look like you in certain spaces or when accessibility is a barrier, it is easy to conclude that it's not meant for you. These are lies, beloved. I invite you to declare what is yours. Know that you are worthy. You're invited to reflect on what might be showing up, any fears that might be germinating, or signs of resistance to integrating yoga as an embodiment practice into your healing journey.

body rites

You are invited to pace yourself in working through the eight themed segments, taking all the time you need with each of them. Each of the eight segments will include moments of holistic self-study, and combination of grounding meditation instructions, breathwork options, and one to three yoga and embodiment shapes/variations. In the 10-week workshop series, we complete the *healing on the mat* journey with West African dance as part of the closing ritual. You're invited to design your own full body movement moment if it feels right.

HERE ARE A FEW TIPS FOR MOVING THROUGH THE WORK |

- Remember the sweet code of healing!
- Go wild with your self-care plan.
- Return to grounding as much as you need to.
- Find a rhythm that works for exploring the activities in this section. You might consider taking a few days in between each theme or maybe a week per theme feels more spacious.
- Listen to your body, beloved.
- If you are working with a therapist, it might feel supportive to your therapeutic work to share what comes up for each of the themes. It's all connected. Your therapist can work through it with you by making it a part of your treatment plan.
- If you have medical conditions or are under the supervision of a physician, you're encouraged to consult as needed regarding physical activity.
- You might begin with the opening ritual you created.
- You are encouraged to read each of the sections one by one, taking time with the writing prompts and self-study and flowing through the healing practices at your own pace.
- Remember you can skip and/or unapologetically modify as much as you need to.
- When it feels right, you might try on some of the tools in your daily life.

EMBODIED HEALING |

OK, so when I said this was an embodiment journey, I really meant it, beloved. The invitation and practice of returning to your body, trusting that it knows the truth, and making a home inside of it lives cover to cover. Perhaps you have already been noticing some things about your relationship with your body, how it moves in space, or maybe that you are not noticing much at all. You are right where you need to be, beloved.

When I named my business some years ago now, *embodied truth healing and psychological services*, the word embodiment had not yet become so utilized. It's a strange thing to be having a perpetual experience of something, but for there to not be a common nomenclature for it. This accurately depicts the collective reality of many survivors of sexual trauma who have had traumatic lived experiences that they cannot find words for. Further, those experiences are often disembodying. They take us out of ourselves, out of our bodies. I find it quite logical to want to escape a place that reminds us of our pain, that does not feel safe, that other people do not respect. Our attempts to survive can truly be one of the most vibrant aspects of our creativity. By all means we survive, even if it means being a visitor in own bodies.

I am placing flowers at your feet.
I pray that if you can see them, you will know that you are awake.
If you can smell them, you will know that you are here now.
I pray that you will pick them up and hold them close to your body,

That you will thank it for waiting for you (for holding you).

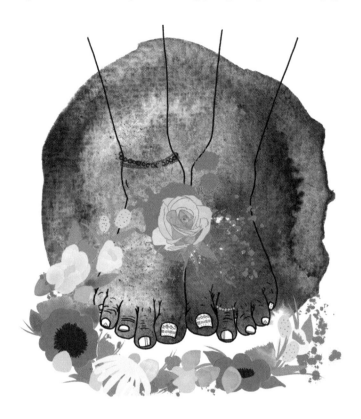

When disembodiment becomes the norm, it can be challenging to sustain sense of presence, to tolerate intense or charged sensations, to notice what's happening in the body, or how the body is moving in space. This can look like frequently losing track of time, mentally zoning out, having moments where your emotions don't match the situation, consuming foods that trigger reactions in your body, or bumping into furniture/doors often.

body rites

You're invited to cozy up with your workbook and write your reflections in the space held below.

What are you wondering or feeling curious about in what you are reading?

What sensations are you noticing in your body in this moment?

How does your body show and tell you what it's been through?

What do you remember about your body before having an experience of sexual trauma? How is your body and/or relationship with your body different?

BREATH AS A TOOL |

Breathing can be a way of making intentional contact with yourself to energize or to calm. I invite you to consider how the breath can be used as a focal point that also supports being present. Paying attention to your breath will be a useful companion as we journey forward. Know that there is no requirement for breathing a certain way. You might decide to breathe normally as that might feel most supportive to you. Your choices are celebrated! If it feels right, I invite you to take some time exploring different breathing options.

You might compassionately observe your breath to begin. Just notice what's happening without changing it.

You're invited to circle and write in your observations of what's happening with your breath right now.

Full even breaths

Holding my breath

Short inhalations

Long breaths in

Shallow breathing

Chest rises when I breathe

Tummy moves in and out

Short exhalations

Long breaths out

_____

_____

_____

body rites

- The breath is a masterful teacher. Dropping in to notice what's happening with the breath is also a way of bearing witness to ourselves. It's a great time to be curious. Remembering, constricted inhalations could reflect challenges receiving, while short exhalations might attest to difficulties letting go. And for many of us, we are out here constantly holding our breath, a tell-tale sign of bracing for something bad to happen or being suspended in dread. Similarly, chest breathing often fuels anxiety, while breathing that begins and ends in the tummy activates the parasympathetic nervous system.

- You're encouraged to explore how you might gently bring harmony and balance to your breath, keeping your observations close to your heart. Perhaps by elongating the in and out breath, slowing it down, or asking it to begin and end in the tummy. Stay here as long as you like. You know what's best for you.

- Before you move into embodiment practices, yoga shapes, and meditation, you might take a quick peek inside, noticing what changed, and what stayed the same. If it feels right, jot down some notes and reminders of how you can improve the quality of your breath. These will be good to remember throughout your self-healing journey.

body rites

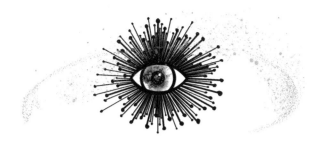

Meditation |

you're encouraged to read through the following meditation guidance in full before beginning.

- To begin you're invited to choose a seated shape, on the floor or on furniture.
- Again, inviting the eyes to make a choice—closing, gazing, or remaining open.
- Connect with the sensation of support underneath your body. If it feels OK, allow yourself to sink into the support for a little while, noticing what that changes in your body.
- If it feels OK, you might explore anchoring into the support while inviting length and spaciousness in the body. You might do this by lifting the crown of the head toward the sky, spreading the collar bones across the chest, melting shoulder blades down the back.
- Observing the breath, you might bring in those reminders of the ways you can bring harmony to the breath—slowing it down, elongating, equalizing.
- Feel into the tummy, expanding on the inhales and deflating on the exhales. You might breathe in something you need and exhale what you don't.
- Remembering the support underneath your body, expanding into space, and allowing the breath to flow through.
- You're encouraged to breathe this way for 10 cycles of breath, if it feels right.
- Once you feel complete, you're invited to pause and notice what changed before reconnecting with the physical space you are in.

Yoga shapes | for grounding + sensing

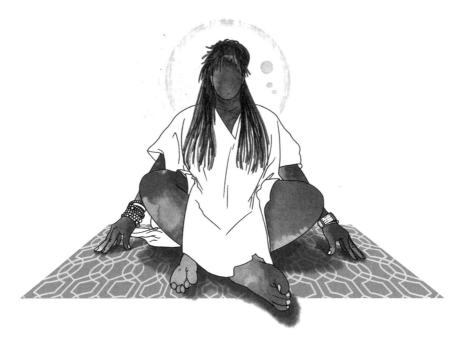

I.   sitting with legs crossed or extended, tent hands with fingertips to the earth, floor, or a surface other than your body (Sanskrit name | sukhasana)

    a)   Notice the sensation of support, of being held up by the earth, floor, or furniture.

    b)   If you're able, you might bring awareness to the fingertips and sensations of stability, stillness, or change in temperature.

    c)   When you gently press into the finger tips, notice what happens with your body and the breath (e.g., does the heart-space open, does breathing become easier or harder?).

    d)   You're encouraged to make any additional adjustments that feel supportive to grounding.

body rites

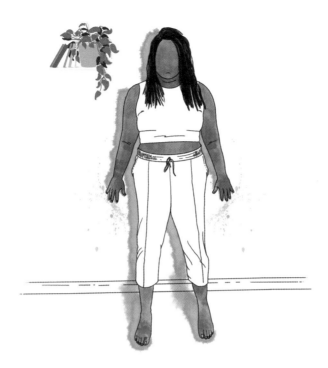

II. sitting or standing with the back of the body against a wall

   a) Notice the sensation of the wall supporting you.

   b) You might bring awareness to sensations of any differences in temperature (e.g., is the wall cold or warm, is it hard or textured?).

   c) When you lean into the wall, notice what happens with your body and the breath.

   d) You're encouraged to explore having the support of the wall feels like, making additional adjustments as you need.

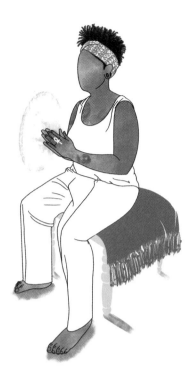

III. rubbing hands together

    a) If you're able, rub your hands together, slow or fast for 20–30 seconds.

    b) Notice the heat building between them.

    c) Gently place both hands somewhere on the body in need of warm self-healing touch (e.g., on the head, heart, tummy, knees, lower back).

    d) Notice what happens with your body and the breath.

    e) Rewarm the hands by rubbing them together and repeat as many times as you'd like.

body rites

BEING A SELF-DEFINER |

I believe self-determination is a path to liberation. The second theme of the *healing on the mat* workshop series is "being a self-definer." It's about remembering and reclaiming your essence, your I AM, deciding who you want to be on the other side of trauma. There are so many layers to cut through here. The weight of expectations placed on you by others, the residue of sexual abuse lying to you about who you are, the influence of individual and collective context, and systemic pressures bullying your self-perception, to name a few. You know the old saying, if you hear something enough, you'll start to believe it. We live in a world that projectile vomits hatred and lies onto Black beings and our bodies. Even though we try to shield and protect ourselves, inevitably some of the lies seep into our pores and mix in with what we know on the inside. For example, I invite you to read the two descriptions below and reflect on experiences you've had that sound similar.

Objectification | roughly defined as seeing and/or treating a person, often a girl/woman, as an object; as lacking autonomy, as something to be owned, and as someone whose experiences/feelings need not be taken into account (Stanford Encyclopedia of Philosophy, 2011).

Sexual objectification | treatment of a person as identified with their body or body parts, in terms of how they look or how they appear to the senses (Stanford Encyclopedia of Philosophy, 2011).

Can you relate?

You're invited to consider times in your life you've been objectified by others, by family members, colleagues, partners/lovers, and/or perpetrators of sexual abuse. What are phrases you've heard often or names that you have been called?

How have experiences of being objectified harmed your sense of self? You're invited to consider various aspects of your identities, e.g., gender, culture, race, etc.

How have other people's expectations/the ways they view you influenced who you have become?

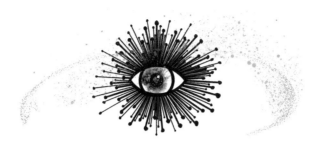

Meditation | focused on I AM . . .

- You're invited to choose a shape, seated or perhaps standing. Whatever you choose is just right.

- Feel into the part of your body touching the earth or floor, growing up from there.

- As you're ready, observe the breath.

- You're invited to explore inhaling breath from that part of you at the earth, allowing it to pass up through the body and exhaling it out of the crown of the head.

- When it feels right, call your attention to your third eye, the space between the eyebrows. If it feels helpful, you might bring one or two fingers to the third eye.

- With every inhale, you're invited to pull the breath in from the earth and with every exhale silently or audibly affirming the truth of who you are by stating I AM _____ and filling in the blank (I AM healing, whole, brave . . .). Stay here as long as you'd like, beloved.

- In time, you might pause to notice the sensations of your affirmations moving through you.

- Guide yourself back into the present and perhaps reconnect with the physical space you're in by noticing a couple of things that have a similar color or shape.

Yoga shapes |

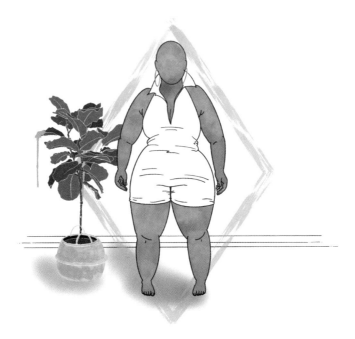

I. mountain pose arms by side/palms forward, hands over heart, or one hand over heart/
    tummy (Sanskrit name | tadasana)

    a) Notice how this shape feels.

    b) Do you feel closer to or farther away from yourself?

    c) How can your breath support you in this moment/shape?

    d) Is there anywhere in your body you can take up more space?

    e) You're encouraged to make additional adjustments or explore any hand/arm place-
        ments that feel right.

body rites

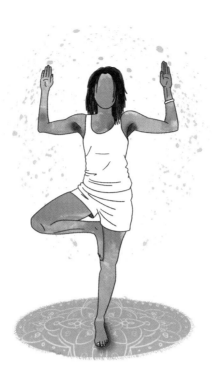

II. tree pose with foot at calf or inner thigh *not on joints,* arms in goal post, extended above the head, or another variation of your choice (Sanskrit name | vrksasana)

    a) Notice how this shape feels. Don't be afraid to use a wall or chair for support with your balance.

    b) How might you embody the energy of a tree in this moment? A tree doesn't ask for permission to take up space. It grows down, and up, and out with fervor and life.

    c) Maybe invite connection with the breath to expand.

    d) You're encouraged to take your time on one side and switch to the other as you're ready, remembering that each side is different and may ask for more of your compassion or patience.

MAKING CHOICES/ADAPTABILITY |

you're doing it, beloved. I'm so proud *with* you. You are making the choice to heal. Often, it is easier to choose what we've known for so long. The self-sabotage, avoidance, being a passenger in our life, looking for chaos. We've all been there, somewhere. I invite you to take some time to share some appreciation for yourself, for returning to the opportunity to heal, for choosing to BE in the driver's seat.

> *It's as if in these moments our bodies don't belong to us*
>
> *And it's as if after those moments*
>
> *Our bodies don't remember*
>
> *Who they belong to.*

The third theme of *healing on the mat*, making choices/adaptability, focuses on the connection between experiences of sexual trauma and difficulty making choices for our bodies. Choice is medicinal, beloved. You've already made so many choices on this journey. We will continue in that flow, with more intentional moments to practice making small, manageable choices for your body and more curiosity about the places choice gets choked by fear, helplessness, and uncertainty.

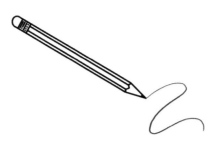

How has being sexually violated impacted your ability to make decisions for

Yourself?

Your body?

Your relationships?

All these things considered, setting and maintaining holistic healthy boundaries can be quite challenging. A boundary—emotional, physical, sexual, energetic, or spiritual—clarifies how much access you are consenting to and also gives you permission to be unavailable altogether.

How do you know when others are violating your boundaries?

What does it feel like in your body when it happens?

What challenges arise when setting and holding boundaries?

You're invited to reflect and write in 1–2 boundaries for each of the categories below. Reference the examples for inspiration as you'd like. Know that you are supported in growing this list of boundaries over time, in healing.

body rites

Emotional

Inspo: please ask if I am in a space to listen before sharing with me.

- _____
- _____

Physical

Inspo: please do not comment on my body/weight.

- _____
- _____

Sexual

Inspo: I am not comfortable having sex in that position, let's try something else.

- _____
- _____

Spiritual

Inspo: I appreciate you trying to understand rather than change or critique my spiritual views.

- _____
- _____

Digital

Inspo: I am not comfortable with you following me on social media and liking my posts.

- _____
- _____

Someone(s) stole your choice when they decided for you

They took your body into their own hands and out of yours

And with it you may have watched your voice trail behind

Or felt it become lodged in your throat, skewered by your breath

You may have seen the sense of where your body begins and ends dissolve

The choices are medicinal, beloved

May you choose healing in every moment

May you choose to snatch yourself back

Hold it like it belongs to you

Hold on to you and your body

Hear your voice return, singing musical YESes and NOs

Feel your breath be free and wild

In your body, where you belong.

Meditation |

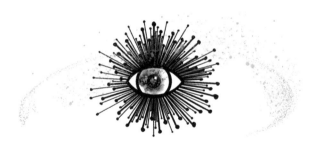

- Settle into a shape of your choice, seated or lying down perhaps.
- Remember the ground is there.
- Allow the eyes to make a choice.
- Begin observing the breath when you're ready.
- You're encouraged to gently make adjustments to the breath that feel supportive.
- You might explore breathing in from the tummy, guiding the breath up to the lungs and chest on the inhale, turning the breath over like an ocean wave, exhaling chest–lungs–tummy.
- When it feels right, explore your edges, the bounds of your physical body; noticing if they are soft, hard, textured, well formed, or porous. Noticing if finding your body's edges with your mind's eye comes with ease or if it requires more effort.

body rites

- You might explore tracing the edges of your body with your mind's eye or by physically tracing your edges with light or firm touch.

- Perhaps an affirmation rises up, (e.g., *"I am here in this body, this is my body, my body belongs to me."*). You're invited to repeat this to yourself, silently or audibly. If you're able, it might feel right to bring the hands to the heart or one hand to the heart, one to the tummy.

- Take all the time you need here.

- Notice what changed and what didn't change.

- Guide yourself back into the present when you're ready, maybe taking a moment to appreciate something in your physical space.

Embodiment shapes |

I. You're invited to describe/draw what your body feels like when you are shrinking/compromising your boundaries.

   a) Once you've identified the shape, you're invited to try it on by bringing your body into that position.

   b) Notice any sensations or emotions that come up.

   c) What's happening with your breath?

   d) You're invited to shift out of this shape when you are ready in whatever way feels right.

II. You're encouraged to describe/draw a shape your body creates when you are feeling assertive and confident.

a) Once you've identified the shape, you're invited to try it on by bringing your body into that position.

b) Noticing any sensations or emotions that come up.

c) What's happening with your breath?

d) Is this a shape that you want to shift out of quickly or stay in longer?

INTUITIVE HEALING & SPIRITUALITY |

In my experience and in witnessing many, I have noticed what I might consider one of the most detrimental wounds/obstructions of sexual trauma—the wound to a relationship with

body rites

our intuition. Not knowing where our intuition lives in our bodies and not being able to recognize the voice or feeling of it. For some of us, likely because we have found some illusion of safety outside of our bodies, it may even be tricky to differentiate the familiarity of trauma misleading you and your intuition guiding/warning you. I invite you to pause and check in with yourself. Am I telling your story?

The fourth theme of healing on the mat, *intuitive healing and spirituality*, is my favorite of the series. It feels like a magical remembering. It's deep deep, beloved. How would things be different if we were raised to trust our intuition? What if our caregivers, in addition to saying "trust your gut," had a practice of nurturing it and cultivated an environment for true intimacy with our inner voice and spirit when we were little ones. How would life be different?

> *Our intuition is a vessel for our higher self, ancestors,*
> *and spiritual guides to speak to us.*
> *In being able to sense into our intuition with clarity*
> *and being able to differentiate it from our traumas,*
> *we access a deeper knowing in our bodies and spirits.*

There's another few layers to peel back here. Earlier, I talked about how sexual trauma at any point in life can obstruct relationship to the Spirit. I've sat with many survivors who say things like "if there was a God, how could he/she/they allow this to happen to me?" Or of whom had a vibrant spiritual practice before, and after can't seem to bring themselves to pray or connect in ways that were at one time fulfilling. There's something about this type of trauma that rubs us so raw, makes us believe we are alone, and squelches the fire in our spirit. This is an elusive reality to live in.

I've discovered that when we invite spirit and intuition into our healing, we can R E M E M B E R. The rawness can create an opening. An opening to remember what was lost or forgotten. Black beings are constantly navigating the wounds of oppression and degenerative conditioning. And in the spiritual aspect, we have been trained to externalize our intuitive process, to color within the lines, and to exist on autopilot. The rawness can create an opening to remember. Remember our kinship to the lands, the elements, the cosmos, our ancestors, creator, and all that guides us. We will be exploring this more throughout the healing journeys that follow.

The rupture

Experiencing sexual trauma can compromise the relationship between a survivor and connection to intuition. For example, as a little one, having the feeling that what was happening wasn't OK, but was told otherwise, perhaps by being made to feel special. That little being may grow up doubting their intuition and inner wisdom. Or as an adult being coerced and pressured into saying yes with your mouth, despite your body screaming no. This can lead to confusion and clouded intuitive sense and the feeling of being split between pleasing others and betraying yourself.

The confusion

The way that trauma lives in the body and the sensations of intuitive signaling can be especially difficult to differentiate as they might feel similar. In some moments, the sensations and familiarity of trauma can even evoke a sense of nostalgia or feelings of deja vu. The past may seem to visit us in the present, inspiring sudden strong feelings that cloud our decisions. The immortal aspects of sexual trauma and our intuition speaking to us might produce similar body sensations—warmth, butterflies, or racing heart. This might look like being drawn to people that remind you of someone that hurt you because they feel "comfortable or familiar." It's deep deep, beloved.

Am I telling your story?

Is there anything you'd like to offer yourself in this moment? A moment to breathe, a minute to ground, a pause outside in fresh air, a good cry? Take all the time you need and come back when it feels right.

I trust your intuition.

What are some of your earliest memories/messages received about intuition?

How did sexual trauma negatively impact connection with your intuition?

How do you know when your intuition is speaking to you? What does it sound or feel like? What are some of the sensations of your intuition communicating?

How has your experience(s) of sexual trauma negatively impacted your spiritual life, practices, beliefs?

How has your spirituality supported your healing?

One of the tools I encourage survivors to use in repair of intuition and spirit, is creation and practice of ritual. "Rituals make us no longer passive beings in the cosmos, but we become creative agents of existence" (Mbiti, 1975). These are the spiritual practices we implement in our lives that support spiritual growth, intimacy, divination, and manifestation. In African spiritual traditions, sacred smoke/aromatics, libations, ancestral reverence, drumming and dance, and relationship with Orisha, and rituals offer support in healing, development of our character, and fulfillment of our destiny.

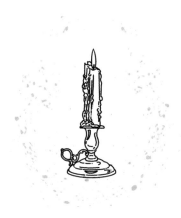

You might feel inspired to create/revisit 1–3 healing rituals. Trust your intuition, beloved. You know just what you need, in spirit. I've listed some ritual inspo, in case it's helpful.

Whispering a sweet prayer into your cup of water, tea, or coffee in the morning

Using a sacred smoke/herb to clear your physical space

Taking a salted bath at the end of the day

Writing for 11 minutes at the beginning of your day

Stretching or doing joyful movement at the end of the work day

body rites

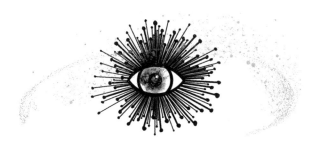

Meditation |

- As you're ready, choose a shape for your meditation practice. If it's a familiar shape, you might explore taking up more space in it. If it's a new shape, maybe you can be curious about what it has to offer.

- Maybe the eyes are ready to make a choice.

- Once you've settled in, begin observing the breath and making any intuitive adjustments that feel supportive. How can you partner with your breath to bring more ease or presence in the moment?

- You're invited to explore inhaling through the nose and exhaling out the mouth.

- When you're ready, I invite you to begin searching for your intuition. Search for where it lives in your body, maybe placing your hands there. If you have trouble locating your intuition this time, that's OK, it may take some time. You're encouraged to be here for about 10 breaths.

- As you breathe, you might ask your intuition to guide you. You can practice repairing the relationship with your intuition by asking yourself in the moment, "what am I feeling?" and "what do I need?" Pausing to listen for the answers. Your needs matter, beloved.

- Guide yourself back into the present, maybe taking a moment to express gratitude to your intuition for its wisdom.

- You're encouraged to take some time to give yourself what's needed, returning when you're ready to practice the following breathing exercise.

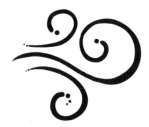

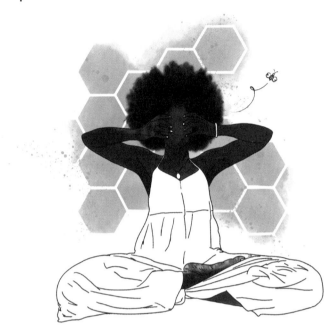

bee's breath two variations |

bee's breath also known as bhramari pranayama, can help minimize the distraction of exter-nal stimuli/noise by redirecting the senses inward and soothe the nervous system. Various mudras (hand gestures that activate/connect with the body's energy in specific areas of the body) will be offered to explore.

- You're invited to find a comfortable seated position.
- *Option 1*
  - Take a full in breath through the nose and out breath through the mouth as you're ready. Connect with a flow of inhalations/exhalations through the nose.
  - Allow the eyes to make a choice.
  - If you're able, bring the index fingers to the cartilage right at the opening of the ears, gently applying pressure. You might imagine that you are creating a quiet cocoon for yourself.
  - Find your pace, slowly inhaling through the nose, bringing the tip of the tongue to softly touch the roof of the mouth. On the exhale, hum with the lips closed (as if you could hum the sound/vibration of a buzzing honey bee).
  - You're invited to continue this way for about 5–7 breath cycles.
  - Release the mudra. You're encouraged to observe any sensations in the body, noticing any shifts.
- *Option 2* (illustrated above)
  - Take a full in breath through the nose and out breath through the mouth as you're ready.

Connect with a flow of inhalations/exhalations through the nose.

- Allow the eyes to make a choice.

- If you're able, bring the thumbs to the cartilage right at the opening of the ears, gently applying pressure; index fingers just above each eyebrow pointing toward one another, middle fingers lightly on top of the eyelids, ring fingers resting outside nostrils (careful not to plug the nostrils, you gotta be able to breathe, fam!), and pinky fingers at the corners of the mouth. The fingers placed in each of these areas minimize sensory intake in each respective location.

- Find your pace, slowly inhaling through the nose, bringing the tip of the tongue to softly touch the roof of the mouth. On the exhale, hum with the lips closed (as if you could hum the sound of a buzzing honey bee).

- You're invited to continue this way for about 5–7 breath cycles.

- Release the mudra. You're encouraged to observe any sensations in the body, noticing any shifts.

Yoga shapes |

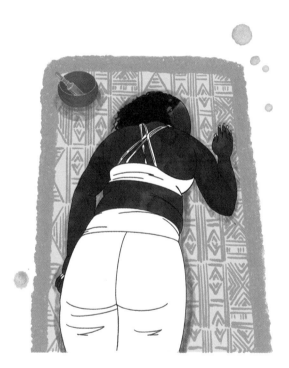

I. laying tummy down forehead to earth, alternating left ear down then right ear

   a) Begin noticing how this shape feels as you are ready.

   b) Notice any sensations or emotions that arise.

   c) Bring awareness to the breath as you can, make any intuitive adjustments.

   d) You might consider exploring the shape, listening for your inner voice until it feels right to either explore placing one ear to the ground and then the other.

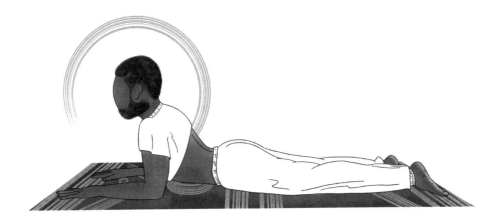

II. sphinx pose (Kemetic name | heru amkhet / Sanskrit name | salamba bhujangasana, niravalasana)

 a) Notice how this shape feels as you settle in.

 b) Gently observe any sensations or emotions.

 c) Spend time connecting with the breath as a support if you'd like.

 d) Maybe explore any ways to also connect with what the shape has to offer you.

 e) You're invited to shift out of this shape when you are ready in whatever way feels right.

body rites

NURTURANCE |

When was the last time you hugged yourself?

I am so inspired by you. You keep showing up and you are so worth it. You are worthy of experiencing joy and peace in your body. This theme of nurturance sets a tone for understanding how you nurture and love yourself and also any tendencies of neglect, self-harm, and shame. As you explore and search yourself, I encourage you to practice self-compassion throughout.

What does it mean to nurture something?

In what ways do you nurture yourself?

Others?

Which feels easier and why?

Our earliest examples of nurturing and caretaking are often parents and caregivers. We literally learn how to care for ourselves (or not!) and others from families of origin and cultural norms. Black beings have a unique history with experiences of caretaking and nurturance, as our enslaved ancestors were forced to care for white people as a means of survival. By any means necessary, we have survived. It is complex though; complicated histories of survival,

body rites

distorted definitions of love, and forced acts of nurturance have informed our individual and collective perceptions of care. These stories—passed down in our bloodlines/DNA, familial patterns/relationships, and communication styles—are alive.

There is immense beauty in these legacies, and also they are laced with pain and shame. We have been conditioned to take care of others first, at the expense of ourselves, and are calling this love. It ain't love fam. It's survival and it's antiquated. Inherently, this pairs well with self-harm and neglect. While we're at it, let's throw a little shame into the mix, we have been in companionship with it for generations. It's not your fault.

Even in this moment, beloved, I invite you to feel into yourself. What do you need right now?

In what ways do you harm or neglect yourself?

Is there any connection between how you harm/neglect yourself and your experience of sexual trauma?

I do hope you are holding yourself with tenderness in your discoveries. Is it true that you don't have to just survive anymore, beloved? Can you live now? When I think about love and nurturance, I'm often brought to my relationship with *little Shena*, my inner child. She is the sweetest being I have ever known, profoundly loving, intensely affectionate, vibrant, and innocent. I am constantly learning from her. I am raising a free, Black inner child. I'm inviting you to reimagine your relationship with your inner child. How can you raise them to live? How can you hold space for their feelings? How can you hold space for them to freely experience pleasure and joy?

Inner child.
A part of us that is always present. That sees all and perhaps feels all.
A part with its own wounds. A teacher. A little one yearning for play.
The best in each of us. The one that needs the deepest love in each of us.

body rites

What are some ways you can nurture and play with your inner child? You're invited to write a list. If it feels OK, you might tap into some of your brightest childhood memories as inspiration.

What are some specific actions/ways you can practice love and compassion with the current version of yourself?

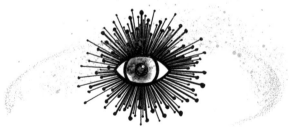

Meditation |

- As you're ready, choose a comfortable shape—seated or lying down.
- You might bring comfort items close—blankets, pillows, a favorite stuffed animal.
- Take your time settling into your shape and the moment, beloved.
- You might ask your eyes how they want to be.
- Connect with your breath, noticing what it needs, what you need to breathe with spaciousness. Maybe there's a breathing technique from a previous section that's calling you.
- When it feels right, bring your inner attention to your third eye. As you reflect on ways to offer more care, nurturance, and play, maybe begin imagining that you are having a visit with a younger version of yourself. You might observe and listen with compassion to what they share,

what they name as needed, the intuitive wisdom they speak. You're encouraged to respond in kind with any intuitive messages, affirmations, or gestures. As you're ready, bring your visit to a close in whatever way feels true.

- Gently guide yourself back into the present, perhaps making physical contact with something in your space that has texture.

- You're encouraged to pause, holding space for yourself and any sensations or emotions surfacing.

Healing shapes |

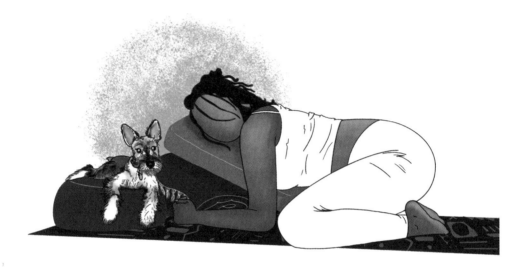

I. commonly referred to as wisdom or child's pose. In African spiritual traditions there is another variation, forehead to the earth shape, as an option. In this variation, the hips are higher than the head. (Sanskrit name | balasana/Yoruba name | moforíbalẹ)

    a) Notice how this shape feels.

    b) You might explore bringing the forehead to the earth/floor, if it feels alright. It's OK if the hips rise, it may feel like a seesaw connection between your head and hips. A pillow underneath the hips is a great supportive option. The illustration above shows a restorative/supported child's pose variation with the torso resting on stacked blankets/pillows.

    c) If it feels OK, on the exhales you might empty any unhelpful thoughts/untruths out of the head and into the earth.

    d) Of course, you don't need permission to adjust your experience in the shape as it feels right. Stay as long as you'd like.

body rites

CONNEXION & KINSHIP |

We've likely never met, and yet I feel so close to you, connected to you in survivorship and in spirit. When the heart is wounded from sexual trauma, no matter the age(s) of occurrence, our relationships can suffer. *Connexion & kinship* is an invitation to explore themes of mistrust, betrayal, and alienation.

Sexual trauma is a relational, interpersonal trauma—something horrific and violating that happens between humans. Inevitably, there is bruising to the heart and relationships. This type of betrayal can impact a person's sense of connection to self and others and can make it tough to trust and engage intimately with others. While this is a reasonable and natural consequence to being unfathomably hurt, it can lead to tendencies to isolate or avoid vulnerability. This can also contribute to choosing relationships that mimic familiar pain.

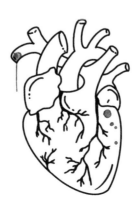

How has experiencing sexual trauma negatively impacted your relationships and sense of connection to others?

How has sexual intimacy been affected?

What barriers or fears do you experience in being vulnerable with others, family, friends, lovers, partners?

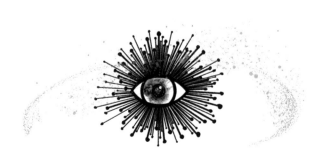

Compassion evaluation |

You're invited to do a compassion evaluation of your closest friendships and relationships, taking a moment to consider how your circle is meeting your support needs, where there is space to ask for more/clarify what you need, and perhaps to consider the possibility of relationships that are no longer serving you.

Who's in your circle?

How is each relationship serving you/what are the strengths of the relationship?

How could they grow/weaken?

What would you like to share with your circle about what you've learned so far about yourself?

What would you like to share (with your circle) regarding what you've learned about your relationships?

What would you like to share regarding what you've discovered about your boundaries?

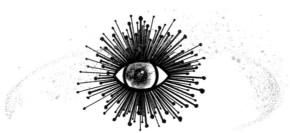

Meditation | heart healing + self-love

- As you're ready, choose a shape, beloved.

- Feeling into the support beneath you, you might notice the temperature or form of whatever is holding you up.

- You might notice that your body and breath are telling you how they want to be for your meditation. You know what's best for you.

- Once you've settled in, you might bring your focus to your third eye. Maybe imagining that you can take a peek down at your heart from the inside. Noticing how it's being, beating, any colors, images, feelings, or textures that show themselves. It's OK to feel how you feel. If the heart had a voice, what would it say to you in this moment?

- You're invited to place one or both hands over the heart space, if it feels right. You might explore massaging the heart space, making circular movements with the palm(s) of the hand, swaying the body side to side, or rocking back and forth. Be here with your heart as long as you'd like.

- When it feels right, check in with your inner vision once more and notice if anything about the heart has shifted.

- Take your time returning to the present moment. You might decide to identify two sounds you can hear or feel the vibration of in or near your physical space.

body rites

Yoga shapes |

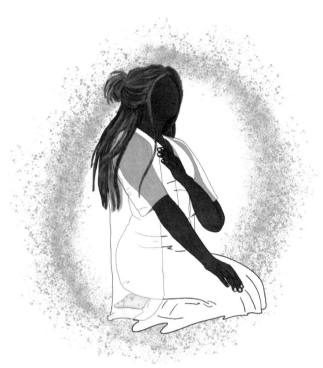

I.   seated hero hand over heart or goal post arms (Sanskrit name | virasana)

a)   Begin to notice yourself in this shape when you're ready.

b)   You might explore placing your hands on your heart, if you're able, or creating a goal post with your arms. You might feel drawn to try both, gently bringing awareness to the sensations of your heart underneath the hands or the heart opening.

c)   As it feels right, observe the breath; you know what to do here to bring flow into your breathing.

d)   It may be helpful to invite in that oceanic breath beginning in the tummy, traveling up to the lungs and chest, and turning it over like a wave on the exhale—chest, lungs, and back into the tummy.

e)   Take as much time as you'd like here.

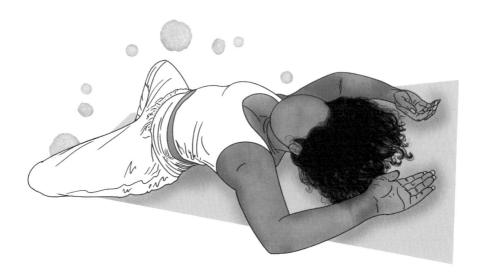

II. person in restorative heart opening butterfly pose (Sanskrit name | supta baddha konasana)

  a) Take your time easing into this shape, beloved. You might consider placing a bolster or pillow underneath the spine and reclining over it for the restorative option, adding extra comfort with a blanket over your body if you'd like.

  b) Notice any sensations or emotions arising. How can you support yourself in this moment? Is there anything you'd like to change (e.g., straightening the legs, placing a pillow/block underneath the knees/legs in butterfly, changing the position of the arms/hands)?

  c) You might observe what's happening with the breath. When you're ready, invite the breath to hold you in any way that feels right.

  d) If it feels OK, maybe you can offer yourself an intuitive affirmation or healing reminder by saying it out loud or whispering it internally.

  e) You might notice what has changed and what hasn't changed since you began your practice today before shifting your shape as you'd like.

body rites

STRENGTH & POWER |

You're a real one, beloved. Healing is possible, and you are putting in so much work. I like to fantasize about Black beings everywhere holding this book, journaling and drawing on its pages, and feeling more like themselves and loving more on each other. It's a powerful dream to imagine, that we are choosing our healing and in doing so our relationships with each other change too. The second to last theme of *healing on the mat* is *strength & power*, but it may be different than what you're thinking.

I remember hearing the words "strong Black woman" commonly threaded together as a young girl. I was raised by the women in my family, a single mother, my older sister, and a club of aunties. I didn't lack examples of what I understood *strongblackwoman* to mean as a little one. There was a palpable sense of pride, of being indestructible, of making it happen by any means necessary. The innuendos were always present; Black women can't afford to be weak, to make mistakes, or to be dependent on anyone, to name a few. I struggle to recall spontaneous expressions of vulnerability outside of funerals. This is not to say that they didn't happen, perhaps this was a "grown-up conversation" or something dealt with in private. I felt that many of the women in my family massaged their grief, sadness, fatigue, disappointment, loneliness, and moments of hopelessness with the down swing of the blues, original R&B, and soul music. Sometimes, I would see tiny pools in one of my aunt's eyes as she sang along to a blues song about a broken heart, or a cousin whose favorite song at Christmas time was about "the lonely." I didn't have the stories, but I caught the vibes.

What messages/examples have you received about being strong? You might consider cultural and gendered influences if it feels right.

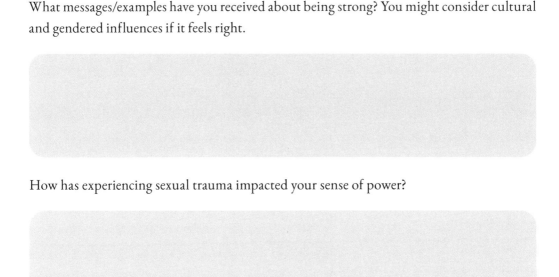

How has experiencing sexual trauma impacted your sense of power?

For Black beings, particularly folks that identify as Black women, being strong is covert for be infallible, defy the odds against you, do it all (gracefully) and quietly, don't complain, and don't you dare show weakness. We are indeed super-human, but we are human, first and foremost. And, we are some of the most traumatized humans on this planet. And also we are transcendent. What would it look like if we rejected the expectations and definitions of strength forced upon us and began to reconstruct ways of being that center our humanity, affirm power in our vulnerability, and that burn the veil of coping in secrecy. Trauma comes in numerous forms, as does coping; but given the wound to the heart, sexual trauma can be especially harmful to our expressions of vulnerability. The guards go up, the armor goes on, and vulnerability can become a friend you once knew or perhaps one you've never known. This is a space to reclaim. An experience you are deserving of. To feel tenderness in your body and to choose to share closeness with those you trust. Vulnerability is kindred to strength.

body rites

What's the difference between conscious vulnerability and passive vulnerability? What do each of these look like in your life/feel like in your body? You're invited to list examples of each, if you'd like.

How can being consciously vulnerable add to your life or experience of support?

What body sensations accompany moments of feeling powerful?

Meditation |

- When you're ready, choose a shape that feels right for your meditation. You might consider choosing a shape that supports being in the energy of power or vulnerability, or perhaps one that allows you to embody both at the same time.

- Once you've settled into the shape, ask your eyes to make a choice.

- Observe the breath, noticing what it wants to reflect for you.

- Begin inviting the breath into the moment when it feels right. To bring coolness to the body you might inhale through the mouth as if you were drinking through a straw, closing the lips on the exhale. Or perhaps there's another breath option you feel drawn to. You're invited to linger here as long as you'd like.

- When you're ready, with your mind's eye, you might begin to (re)imagine what it looks like to move in your power, to see the shapes your body takes on, to experience the sound of power in your voice and becoming perfume in the air around you. You might also (re)imagine what conscious vulnerability looks like on you and in safe spaces. Stay here as long as you wish.

- Notice what changed and what stayed the same.

- Take your time returning to the present, maybe taking a pause to smell something that brings comfort.

Yoga shapes |

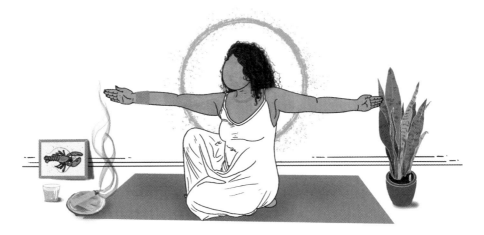

I. Maat Kemetic yoga pose

   a) As you're ready, observe yourself in the shape. Take your time finding a sweet spot.

   b) You might explore accessing your sense of power as you breathe in and out, maybe in through the nose and out of the mouth if it feels right.

   c) Are there any adjustments or variations you'd like to create or explore?

body rites

d) When you're ready, you might try the other side, noticing any similarities or differences.

e) Take your time, shifting out of the shape intuitively.

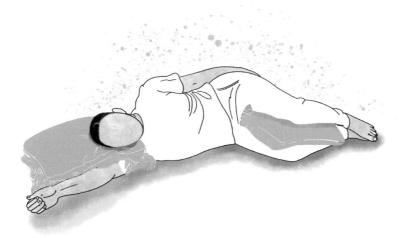

II. side lying shape

a) Notice how this shape feels as you're ready.

b) You might explore placing the knees on either side of a pillow and/or holding a pillow as your little spoon.

c) As you observe any sensations or emotions, you might also check in with your breathing. How can the breath be more supportive to you?

d) If it feels OK, you might imagine a warming of the earth or surface beneath you, on the exhales releasing anything that works against you/peace/presence in this moment.

e) Of course, you don't need permission to adjust your experience in the shape as it feels right. Perhaps roll over to the opposite side if it feels right.

f) Stay as long as you'd like.

BEING WHOLE & AUTHENTIC |

(Be)Whole and Behold, dear one. This is the last theme of *healing on the mat*. I am celebrating with you, every single choice you made to heal, every choice you've made out in the world and in your relationships, every new boundary you've set, every tear shed, every full-bodied YES, and resounding NO you've said, every thing you have reclaimed, beloved. *These are your body rites.* As we wrap up the second journey, we will dive into the practices of wholeness and authenticity, inviting curiosity as to what gets in the way, and closing with an experiment in space and embodiment.

Sexual trauma is fragmenting. It breaks a giant shining star into tiny little pieces, leaving them hanging in the dark. Those pieces of you long and crave to BE together. It can be easy to forget your size, radiance, and wholeness when parts of you are splayed out. It can be tedious to keep track of yourself when you feel broken apart, dulled, hanging in suspension. Oh beloved, you are not broken. Your wholeness is not at stake; you are already whole, you've just forgotten. You are but a beautiful constellation of stars, a milky way, a body twinkling and coming into yourself.

We are not compartmentalized beings. We are full—made of mind, body, heart, and spirit. Surviving asks us to lend this part one way and that part of us another way. To overextend, bend, self-betray, self-sabotage, to empty ourselves, to lose touch with our selves. Beloved, these body rites are a call and response. You do not have to split yourself. You do not have to get by, surviving. You can live, authentically and wholly.

What does authenticity mean to you?

What gets in the way of being authentic?

When is it easiest to be yourself?

When do you feel most whole?

How do you know in your body when you are being your most true self? What does it feel like?

I invite you to take notice, beloved. What has changed and what stayed the same since you began the *body rites* ceremony. You're encouraged to write or draw below.

What do you notice about how your relationship with your body has changed?

How are you different since beginning the *body rites* healing journey?

body rites

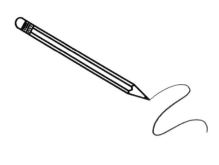

You're encouraged to write yourself a love letter or poem in the space below. The only right way to do it is the way you yearn to do it.

Shapes to be whole and authentic in |

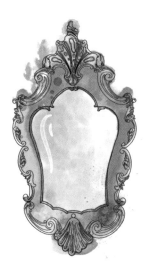

I.

    a)   You're invited to find an uncracked mirror; bring your workbook with you, beloved.

    b)   When you're ready, I invite you to gaze into your reflection; see yourself.

    c)   Noticing any sensations or emotions rising up.

    d)   You might observe your breathing, in your body and in your reflection. Is there anything you can offer yourself to breathe easy?

    e)   When it feels right, you're encouraged to read your poem or love letter out loud. Take your time here, as long as you need.

    f)   You might close this part of the practice with a sweet hug, kissing your reflection, or pressing one of your hands to the mirror if you'd like.

body rites

II.

    a)   It's time to dance, beloved!

    b)   You're invited to choose your favorite healing song or playlist and turn the volume up as loud as your heart desires.

    c)   When you're ready, dance, be free, wild, sensual, whole, and true in your body, in the moment, and beyond.

    d)   Move for as long as you'd like.

shena j young

3rd Journey | *the medicine*

I am beaming. I am moved. My heart is full in journeying with you, beloved. Welcome to the third journey of the *body rites* ceremony. *The medicine* journey, aligns itself with the bottomless opportunity to decolonize healing, to embody your sovereignty, and is an invitation to connect with the energy body and plants/herbs as medicine. Together, we will explore foundational plant/herbal medicine terminology, healing properties, and ways to be in supportive fellowship with them. You'll be encouraged to intuitively try some of the herbal healing practices before we shift into energy medicine. I'll share with you the general anatomy of the energy body, focusing on the seven major energy centers (chakras), their respective psychophysiological and spiritual functions, the African spiritual roots, and the impact of trauma on the chakras. You are in control of what you take in and what you put aside. Know that *body rites* is here for you to come back to as many times as you find yourself returning. I get that healing is densely layered and your workbook is here to meet you where you are. *The medicine* journey will culminate with a holistic practice and collection of rituals, organized by primary energy centers, to flow through at your own pace as always.

As you well know by now, my path as a body-centered psychologist–healer, in many ways, departs from the Westernized concepts that have shaped the field of psychology. It has been an insightful and jarring revelation; that many of the sciences as we know them in the present have African and Indigenous origins. Psychotherapy and psychological theories, archetypal and shadow work ideologies, somatic healing frameworks, and even the chemical formulas used in modern pharmaceuticals have roots in the wisdoms, holistic medicines, and consecrated practices of our African ancestors. I have felt through a range of emotions and resentments about this, that our ancestors were forced to leave their homes and forbidden to practice their traditions only to have these same sacred concepts be reupholstered, appropriated, commercialized, and sold back to us as "revolutionary" or "radical" healing tools. That might be one of the most enduring and oldest forms of gaslighting we've known. Oh beloved, you come from greatness. From people deeply connected to the elements, the cosmos, the Gods, the lands, and the energy of all living beings.

I embody a great sense of pride in knowing this. I offer this background as an anchor for all that I'll be sharing.

I am grateful to have had the courage and humbled by all the subtle plot twists my ancestors orchestrated so that I could do this work as I do. And in doing so, I am effervescently re-membering through them, healing that returns the power to the people. My prayer is that as you continue working through, you will recognize yourself, that your inner wisdom will be illuminated, and that you will catch yourself thinking "I knew that" or "I've wondered about that," and that your relationship with your ancestors is fortified. By no means is what I am sharing in the forthcoming journey intended to be a comprehensive and complete exploration of energy or plant medicine. Rather, I have carefully woven some ideas together that I have collected in my work with survivors of trauma/sexual trauma and the consistent patterns that reveal themselves, time and time again, that may serve as a compass towards embodied healing. In this medicine journey, I continue to draw upon the wisdom I have inherited and channel through my/our ancestors, my teachers in the traditions, my studies, my healing, and all that exists beyond explanation. Remember to trust your intuition, and listen to your body first and always.

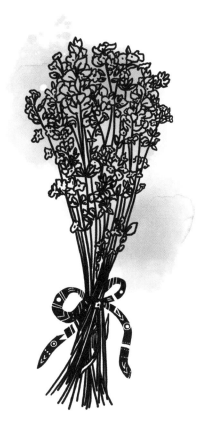

PLANT MEDICINE |

Plants and herbs are elders and ancestors that live among us. They are complex and sacred beings that partner with us in cleansing, nourishing, balancing, adapting, and blessing. They are generous and loyal companions with an enduring capacity to intuitively care for us. I invite you to aim your heart towards the plants so they can recognize you—so they can see generations of your people in the glory of your face, in the gloss of your eyes, in the fullness of your lips.

In many of our ancient lineages and traditions, plants are the roots of medicine. When our dear ancestors were captured, forcefully transported, and enslaved some of the plants were left behind. Thanks to the survival wit of our ancestors, other plants made the journey, hidden on their bodies and tucked away in their crowns. There were many plants that were stolen from their native lands, uprooted, and thrusted into the soil of capitalism. The others deepened their roots in the homeland soil awaiting our return. Welcome to an emboldened return, beloved.

One of my beautiful teachers, xóchicoatl once shared "Plants don't remember colonization in the same way as us. They remember their medicine." While we have had to forget our ways and change ourselves in order to survive, the plant ancestors have held a tight grip on knowing who they are and what they do. They have persisted and thrived, steeping in their potency, despite being called weeds and being demonized. I give thanks to our plant elders and ancestors. Let us all give thanks.

PRAYER FROM XÓCHICOATL |

ometeotl,

with the permission of the four directions, the lands i am with, your corazones and all of your relations, i invite you into prayer. a practice of relating, of remembering, of remembering how to relate, a prayer to connect and move from the power of all of our sacred relations once again.

inviting you to rise, pull back your shoulders, soften your gaze, *breathe in, breathe out.* as we face each gate, allow your heart to open, your sacredness to be (re)membered. we face the east.

sacred direction of the east, house of illumination, bless us with the light of new beginnings. shine your light with clarity and hope on the sacred seed we carry. support us in holding the sacredness we are, and the sacred seeds and dreams we are here to plant. *with humility we offer a word of gratitude, Ometeotl, Àṣẹ.*

breathe in, breathe out, turn

direction of the south we come to you today to remember our guerrere, our warrior. we invite the warriors who came before us to shape our ways. like you, we are here to plant unapologetic, brilliant, and juicy dreams. fill us with the tools, practices, with the courage in each step to live in service of our dream, in service of our sacredness. *with humility we offer a word of gratitude, Ometeotl, Àṣẹ.*

breathe in, breathe out, turn

we turn to the west, where the divine spirits of rebirth emanate. we call on you, sacred medicine of regeneration. support us in transforming and shedding the shadows that keep us from blooming. may we remember that we deserve to bloom. *i deserve to bloom.* they deserve to bloom. and we can bloom together. *with humility we offer a word of gratitude, Ometeotl, Àṣẹ.*

breathe in, breathe out, turn

we come to you great north, resting place of our ancestors to call on our benevolent ones, those who have offered themselves to liberation, to justice, to healing to cycles of violence to walk with us today. inviting you to share your names, your songs, your stories, your ways. inviting you to remind us we never walk alone. *with humility we offer a word of gratitude, Ometeotl, Àṣẹ.*

breathe in, breathe out

we stretch our arms up to the sky, to the celestial gourd above we call on you today to witness us and bathe us in the divine remembering that they are the stars above, we are the stars below and our duty is to shine. bright. *with humility we offer a word of gratitude, Ometeotl, Àṣẹ.*

breathe in, breathe out

body rites

bring yourself to the earth, literally bring your heart down to the earth. we bow our heads to *Tonantzin tlalli, Tonantzin Coatlicue, tierra,* Aye, earth, we come today to remember how to be sacred again. we come to present ourselves to the people of the lands we are on. *if you know the names of the peoples whose lands you occupy, speak to them.* we offer this introduction as a beginning, we come to grow our relation with you, these lands, we come to be in better relation with you. great spirits of the land to teach us how to be generous like earth who offers their back for us to grow our foods and build our homes, their waters so we may not go thirsty, their wisdom so we may always be free. *with humility we offer a word of gratitude, Ometeotl, Àṣẹ.*

breathe in, breathe out

bringing our hands to our heart, we weave to the center. we close this practice here at the center, where all life begins, ends, and connects. here at the center, we ask the spirits of connection, of presence, of remembering we are one. there is no justice for one people, without justice for all, there is no healing for one people, without healing for all. *with humility we offer a word of gratitude, Ometeotl, Àṣẹ.*

xóchicoatl*

(they/she/amor)

HERBAL PREPARATIONS |

xóchicoatl describes herbal preparations as "plant ancestor alchemizations." These are the sacred methods of being in fellowship with herbs, plants, and the medicine they offer. When we bring our healing intentions together with "the body of plant ancestors, waters, liquids, spirits, heat, and the elements," we create living potions that support the physical body and the spirit. There are endless options for working with plants. Most commonly we cook with them, asking for their spice, flavors, and juices to elevate our culinary creations. We add a little of this, a pinch of that. We taste and add more until it's just right. It's second nature.

Our ancestors, African traditions, and Indigenous lineages know the power of herbalism as first nature. To be in community with plants with respect, reverence, gratitude and harmony. We come from traditions where plants and herbs are woven into every life aspect in all life cycles, in cooking and cleaning; for physical, emotional, and spiritual healing; protection; divining; making magic; and so much more. African herbalism entrusts the divinity of plants to "condition the body in its entirety so that disease will not attack it" (Sawandi, n.d., p. 12).

---

* xóchicoatl shares this prayer with the spirit of Caxcan and Wixárika lands, *los montes y vientos* currently holding them. this prayer is rooted in their ancestral traditions of the Mexicayotl, medicine remembered and stewarded by the Mexica people of Mexico. *Ometeotl* is the Mexica guardian of the sacred dual energies, who supports all to live in balance, harmony, and presence in our sacred existence as a being of all.

Plant medicine concoctions were often paired with incantations that protected, freed, and cured the people at the root of the problem (Sawandi, n.d., p. 13). Colonization and capitalism have remarkably severed this intimate relationship. First by restricting access, prioritizing consumption over nourishment, and over time oppressing, abusing, and over-harvesting, only later to extract the medicines, stealing the wisdoms for profit of pharmaceutical formulas. Did you know that one of the main ingredients in one of the most commonly prescribed antibiotic flu medications is a derivative of star anise, an herb? Not only has our herbal wisdom healed our people and lands of the past, it continues to mend us in our present, albeit masked as new technology. Does this sound familiar? Brainwash, steal, oppress, demonize, appropriate, call it an invention or discovery, capitalize, profit, repeat.

In our reclamation, may we restore our relationships with the earth.
May we recognize the likeness in the wounds of violation, ours and the earth's.
May we soften in the shared recognition, in the knowing of each other's stories.
May we take better care of our earth and their medicine, as we heal.

Oh beloved, there is so much to reclaim. My constant prayer and intention is that you are moved to take back your ability to heal yourself. That you root yourself in the consciousness of the healing wisdoms that flow through your blood, that hover in spirit on your back, that coat your intuition, and that honor the truth that you know what's best for you and your body.

There's so much to unlearn and much to evoke in reconnection with African herbalism. This is but a tiny seed among the multitude of medicines. We will be working with three specific herbal preparations for the medicine journey. Herbal tisanes, oils, and baths. You're invited to whisper prayers and healing affirmations to infuse your herbal creations as it feels right. All herbal recipes in *the medicine* journey were lovingly divined by myself and xóchi with thoughts of you and our collective healing at the center. I've shared a description of each herbal preparation on the following pages.

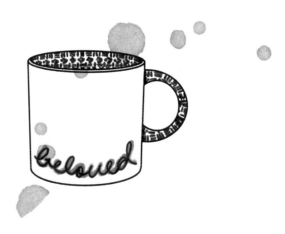

body rites

HERBAL TISANES (TEAS) |

When preparing an herbal tisane or tea, you'll be partnering hot water and herbs (leaves and flowers). Choose a vessel, to which you can add 1–2 tablespoons of herb per cup, or 1–2 teaspoons when working with a more bitter herb. Pour in hot water, cover, and steep for 10–30 minutes (xóchicoatl, 2021, herbal preparations, la mala yerba). Using hot water releases the àṣẹ, or life force energy, of the herbs which is then consumed and offered to the body. If you'd like to go for more of an infusion instead of a tisane, you're invited to steep 4–8 hours or overnight. Naturally, the longer you infuse, the more potent your tea.

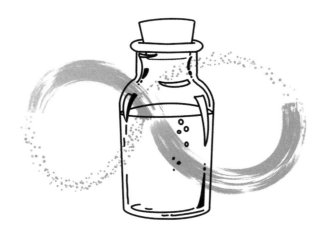

HERBAL OILS |

Herbal oils can be prepared with fresh or dry herbs. I have included recipes that work best with crushed dried herbs for a shorter preparation time as suggested by Dana Woodruff (Woodruff in Scott's Partnering with Plants, n.d., p. 92). If dry herbs are not available, allow the fresh herbs to wilt and dry out as much as possible before working with them. Fill a clean, dry jar halfway with dried (crushed) herbs. Cover herbs with the oil of your choice and poke any air bubbles out with a clean knife. Either place the herbs, ingredients, and oil together in a double boiler or into a metal bowl resting over a pot of water. Very slowly warm the herbs at the lowest temperature as you do not want to cook the herbs in the oil. The intention is to warm them for about 30–60 minutes. Let the oil cool, strain, and then store in an amber or dark bottle. You're encouraged to label your oil including the name of the herb(s), the date, and the healing intention if you'd like.

HERBAL BATHS |

In *Partnering with Plants*, Toi Scott shared an excerpt from Stephanie Rose Bird's *A Healing Grove*, stating in Quimbois culture "many African cultures view the bath tub as a vessel for well-being"; French speaking Caribbean Africans have two primary types of baths, *bain*

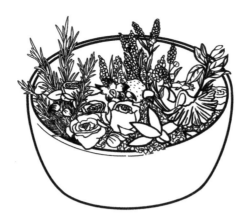

demarre, a bath to get rid of problems, and *bain de la chance,* a bath to bring good luck (Bird, 2009; Scott, n.d., p. 27). In other African diasporic traditions, the bath properties may be classified as bitter or sweet. In the last part of the third journey, you'll be invited to explore an herbal bath and subsequently in the fourth journey a spiritual bath.

In this practice, we ask the herbs to partner with us by cleansing us of negative influences that are impacting our aura or essence (Karade, 1994). To prepare an herbal bath, combine materials in a bowl. Add hot water as you would for an herbal tisane, steep for 10–30 minutes. As you are preparing your herbal bath, you're invited to say a clear prayer of how you would like Spirit to support you. Your words are powerful incantations. Pray fervently for what you need and so deserve.

When sourcing, harvesting, or buying herbal products/materials, please practice mindfulness as many plants are over-harvested, are victims of capitalism, and as a result are nearing extinction. You're encouraged to do your research and seek alternatives for any plants that may be endangered or vulnerable. Choosing to work with apothecaries, botanicas, and companies that locally source, ethically harvest, and maintain fair trade practices are urgently encouraged. I've listed a few things below that might be helpful to have as you journey. As always, they are optional. Working with what you have is an ancient and resourceful choice.

OPTIONAL SUPPLIES |

Various dry or fresh herbs contingent on recipes to follow

Tea pot or boiling pot/saucepan

Double boiler or metal bowl

Strainer or cheesecloth

Small spray bottle (preferably glass, amber or dark colored, or stainless steel)

Glass jar/container (small to medium)

Your favorite tea mug

body rites

"Partnering with plants in a truly reciprocal manner is very powerful. As long as we remain humble, they will continue to teach us and share their healing gifts. They are the true healers and we are a conduit or a vehicle for that healing."

—*Toi Scott, Partnering with Plants, p. 36*

HOW HERBS TOUCH THE BODY |

Our herbal ancestors are made of wisdom, medicine, and time. They have lived for generations and are quite sophisticated in their existence. They belong to plant families that support our nourishment, ability to adapt, to fight, to resist, and to heal. Within their anatomy are the vitamins and minerals that reach in and touch each of our bodily systems, encouraging restoration and more optimal functioning. Before we shift the vibe into energy medicine, I'm inviting you into an intuitive exploration of your relationship with the plant ancestors. Take your time with the following activities. You know more than you know.

WISDOM NOTES | (HERB ACTION GLOSSARY, LA MALA YERBA, XŌCHICOATL, 2021):

Common herb actions helpful to know when healing from sexual trauma

Adaptogenic—guide the body into a state of resistance to stress and support ability to adapt to extraordinary challenges

Analgesic—relieve pain

Blessing—often partnered as sacred smokes, aiding us in neutralizing physical space, clearing negative energy, and/or inviting in spiritual support

Demulcent—have a soothing action on inflammation, especially the body's mucous membranes

Nervine—are soothing and calming to the nervous system

Nutritive—provide vitamins, minerals, and nutrients

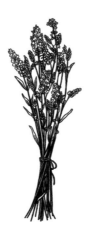

HERBAL PRACTICE |

You're invited to identify 3–5 household herbs that you currently work with, either fresh or dried.

Write them in below and intuitively fill in the chart as labeled. In order to complete the last column, you may need to do some research. Remember this is an intuitive activity. Choose an herb, make some intuitive guesses about its healing properties, and compare your notes with what you discover in your research. I've offered an example below in case that feels helpful.

name of herb	intuitive guesses about its healing properties	researched healing properties
e.g., star anise	clears out toxins, decongestant	antifungal, antibacterial, anti-inflammatory

body rites

Any surprises?

What did you discover?

Choose 3–5 more from the list below, add them to the table, and repeat the instructions above.

cinnamon	chamomile	sweet grass	parsley
garlic	echinacea	ginger	cayenne
rosemary	fennel	licorice	wild yam root
cannabis	lemongrass	basil	lavender

What did you discover?

What herbs on this list might be supportive for you?

energy is a vibe |

"If we are to fully experience spirit, as earthly beings, we need to feel truly embodied; by this I mean at home in the body . . . . The body offers many limitations to embrace, and the spirit offers liberation. Knowledge of the chakra system provides the opportunity for both embodiment—feeling the spirit move in the body—and enlightenment—freeing the life of the body."

—*Caroline Shola Arewa,* Opening to Spirit, *p. 38*

We have likely all had the experience of someone entering a shared space and being turned off by their energy. We might hear ourselves and others say things like "it's hard to be around so and so; their energy ain't right" or after spending time with someone realizing that we feel drained. On the contrary, you may be able to recall an encounter with someone who's energy lights up a whole room, you feel yourself drawn to them, and perhaps you feel energized in having their company. *Energy is a vibe; it's real.* Occasionally (or frequently) you might have the experience of feeling like you need space from others, time in nature, a shower at the end of a work day or after a bad dream. Maybe when you enter a space you can feel that something is off, maybe there's been a conflict or there's lingering tension in the air, or after leaving a family gathering you feel heavy, as if there is an invisible residue sticking to your body. These are just a few examples of how energy exchanges are present in our daily lives.

catch the vibe | an energy meditation

- You're encouraged to read the following instructions entirely before beginning.
- You're invited to choose a comfortable seated shape, feeling yourself held up by the earth or piece of furniture.

- When you're ready, bring your awareness to your breath making any intuitive adjustments that support presence. You might allow the eyes to make a choice, gently closing, softly gazing down, or remaining open.

- As the breath becomes more full, slow, or even, I invite you to consider a color that describes your energy in the moment. Whatever shows up first is often most true. As you hold that color

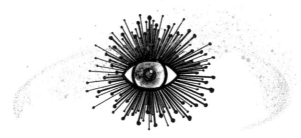

  in your mind's eye, if you're able, begin rubbing the hands together for about a minute. You'll notice that this begins to generate heat between the hands.

- When you're ready, quiet the hands and begin slowly pulling them apart, noticing the sensations and energy present between the hands. You might feel inclined to move the hands closer together and then farther apart, and close together again and so on with alternating distance. Or maybe you experiment with cupping the hands as if you can mold or hold the energy like a ball. Notice any colors or textures that arise. Stay here as long as you'd like.

If you had some difficulty sensing into the energy, not to worry. It can take time to nurture our natural sensitivity and remove the energetic callouses. You might consider taking a break and trying again moving even slower this round or returning to the exercise another time altogether.

WISDOM NOTES |

You may have noticed a magnetic push and pull between the hands.

Maybe the color you identified at the beginning was the same or different than the energy between the hands.

Sensations of heat, tingling, and pins and needles are also possible among others.

Various emotions may also have come up. These can be helpful to simply observe in the moment and instrumental in reflection after.

What did you notice?

Were there any colors or textures that came up? If so, you're encouraged to describe them below.

You're invited to draw a picture of what you experienced, or perhaps an image that represents how you feel in the moment.

body rites

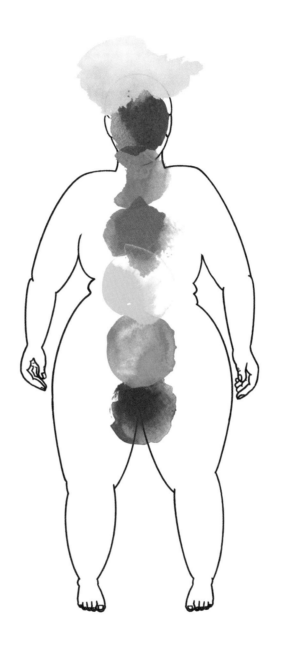

THE ENERGY CENTERS/CHAKRAS |

The energy body speaks a language we all know.

We all have the capacity to sense and work with energy. I come to you here with humility on my path as an energy healer, raised up by my teachers in the Usui reiki lineage (Nayelli Cardenas, Brooke Albrigo, Zel Amanzi), my self-study of wisdom texts (Caroline Shola Arewa, Baba Ifa Karade, Donna Eden), my yogic studies and collage of teachers since 2008, my expansion and adamant return to the source in African spirituality/Yoruba tradition, and the many energy bodies I have been in fellowship and exchange with since I was a little Shena. Mojúbà to the source and motherland, to the African diaspora and its people for creating, carrying, and spreading this ancient energy medicine from so many corners and cultures of the world. Mojúbà to the ancient Egyptians— the people of Kemet, the Yoruba people, the Indus-Kush people, their descendants, and all of us—the multigenerational heirs of rich medicinal wealth. Àṣẹ.

The energy body anatomy is meticulously woven throughout and just beyond our physical being. The energy body consists of the aura, a multilayered personal energy field, the minor, major, and minute chakras, and the energy pathways known as meridians or nadis (Arewa, 1998, p. 5–6). We will focus on the seven major energy centers (root, sacral, solar plexus, heart, throat, third eye, and crown), their functions, and the impact of trauma as a continuation of the *body rites* healing ceremony.

Chakras, derived from the Sanskrit language of India, means "wheel" and are swirling, vibrating *energy centers* or vortices each positioned at one of seven points along the spine to the top of the head and numerous throughout the body. In addition to having the ability of spinning clockwise and counterclockwise, "Your chakras pull their energy in from your environment (including, for better or worse, the energies of other human beings) and distribute them in your body. Your chakras also send energy outward" (Eden, 2008, p. 158). The chakras are quite magical and powerful in all the ways they touch our being and existence. Caroline Shola Arewa reminds us that "the chakras unite us with our Ancestors, who bestow blessings upon us. The wisdom of past, present, and future is revealed to us via the chakras" (Arewa, 1998, p. 4). They have three overarching functions—physiological, psychological, and spiritual—that support our development, well-being, and consciousness. Optimal functioning, harmony, and embodiment of the chakras respective themes/tasks help us to live in our wholeness. When there is disharmony, impaired energies, blockages, or stagnancy in any of the chakras, physical health issues and dis-ease, mental health challenges, somatic symptoms, and spiritual aimlessness are inevitable.

body rites

We have galaxies of healing wisdom in our bodies, beloved. I like to relate to each energy center as its own planet within a larger energetic solar system. Each chakra is its own intricate world with a unique constellation of characteristics, special connection to the elements, lands, and planets, and most importantly its divine soul task/intention. Just as the solar system orbits and communicates among the planets, the moon, sun, and stars, so do our chakras. The first three relating to our inner self/inner reality, the fourth the bridge and alchemy center hosting our transformation, and the other three shift into our higher self/divine reality. The chakras are independent and interdependent in their respective responsibilities and in the culture and communication between them. Ideally, our energy centers are radiantly spinning, actualizing in their soul tasks, and in an emanating flow of constant communication with one another. However, life can be complicated, and when it impresses upon our energy body—our chakras in particular—disharmony in one chakra can eclipse the vitality and effective mechanics of the others.

You're invited to pause for a moment, breathing in all of this remembrance, and exhaling sending it into your energy body. You might take 5–7 breaths inhaling the ancient wisdom, perhaps as a color or sound, and exhaling for integration and recognition in your body. Take as long as you need here.

You might also consider making some notes about what is coming up for you as you progress through the material. What's resonating? What feels familiar? Are you noticing any resistance? What's lighting you up? You might also check in with your body and notice if you are experiencing sensations of contraction or expansion. Trust yourself in giving your body what it needs.

THE IMPACT OF TRAUMA ON THE CHAKRAS |

"Memory is energetically encoded in your chakras just as it is chemically coded in your neurons . . . . An imprint of every important or emotionally significant event you have experienced is believed to be recorded in your chakra energy . . . "
—*Donna Eden and David Feinstein,* Energy Medicine, *p. 147*

In a body moving through life, collecting stories, and making connections, the energy centers are its *griots*. In African lineages, the griots hold a highly regarded position in community. They are the historians, the storytellers, the vocalists, cultural performers—the griots keep the stories alive. The chakras are our bodies' griots, archiving our stories, sharing and storing them throughout our energy body, our organs, glands, and various bodily systems. Naturally, lived experiences and stories of peace and joy charge our physical and energy beings with goodness, while harboring traumatic experiences drain and cause erosion from the inside out. Any important or emotionally significant events are recorded in the chakras as energy memory (Eden, 2008). Just as our life memories are encoded in our brains, our lived experiences are imprinted on our chakras. This is not to say that every memory stored in our brains or in our chakras are ones that we are able to recall vividly in our minds. The body is quite sophisticated in its mechanisms of protection.

body rites

Certainly, it is possible, as I mentioned in so many words earlier, that we can have body memory for something that we don't remember. This holds true in the realm of energy too. Our energy memory and consciousness are not necessarily reading from the same page, despite being in the same body. Considering the impact of trauma on the energy centers can be especially revealing. In imagining, reflecting, and exploring the imprint of traumatic experiences on our chakras, we can gain clarity about personal, psychological, physical, and spiritual challenges. Trauma stored as energy memory can directly affect the chakras' ability to support us in their respective soul-task or function as they often become blocked, or over- or under-stimulated. Energy memory extends beyond life in the body you have now, and often or likely tells the stories of previous lifetimes, yours and those of your ancestors. Just as our ancestors' stories are infused in our DNA and blood, they are also imprinted on our chakras. Deep deep, right?

Because the chakras and energy memory are intricately unique and personal, there is not a universal manifestation of trauma. However, there are a few common patterns. The chakra(s), in its over-/under-stimulation or due to blockages:

- is not optimally able to achieve its soul-task/intent
- may not be able to effectively support its respective physiological, psychological, or spiritual functions
- will be cut off from communication with other chakras, affecting the overall flow of energy and ability to transcend

As you might imagine, this can inspire a number of holistic complications. In my work with survivors of trauma, there have been some consistent patterns as well. Keep in mind, our framework—that trauma affects us mind, body, heart, and spirit. As you read through the following list, I encourage you to make mental notes of resonance with your experience or perhaps those of your loved ones. These descriptions are not exclusive to survivors of sexual trauma, although I will also highlight those that are most prevalent in my work with survivors. Here are a few of the general possibilities.

- Increase in physical health issues/symptoms
- Bouts of depression and/or anxiety or other psychological symptoms
- Repressive tendencies, pushing down feelings/experiences in order to not deal with them
- Disconnection from spiritual realm and higher self

Ultimately, instead of optimal function of the energy center, there is dys-function and inversion of the soul task. For example, the heart chakra's soul task is love, relating, and compassion. The impact of trauma could express in themes of resentment and depression, psychologically and as hypertension, physically. In my work with survivors of sexual trauma, the 1–3 energy centers are pervasively compromised and imbalanced, which makes sense given how violating sexual trauma is to the sense of self. Often, this is where our work begins while also affirming evidence of disharmony in the heart and the 5–7 energy centers. This is likely not shocking to you beloved, although it may be generating a web of connections; perhaps to some of the themes that came to light in your first two journeys. I invite you to take some time and be with what's coming forward.

What's your intuition telling you? As you are reading and processing about the impact of trauma on the chakras, what intuitive guesses or senses do you have about which of your seven major energy centers might be imbalanced, blocked, or stagnant? How do you know? (It may be helpful to turn back to view the figure at the beginning of the energy section on p. 101.)

Which energy centers would you guess or feel are open and balanced? What gives you this sense?

THE PRACTICE |

How are you feeling, beloved? Do you ever ask yourself that and actually answer, sincerely? How are you feeling and what do you need? I encourage you to tend to you with some tenderness, if it feels right. You've been taking in and remembering so much. We've journeyed up to *the medicine practice*. These body rites are yours to claim, to pass through on the way home. When you're ready, I've offered some notes of preparation and guidance below. Please know, as always, your way *is* the best way and your choices are supported.

The medicine journey will guide you through a practice with each of the seven major energy centers. Given the natural relationship between the chakras, it is suggested to flow in order from the root to the crown. *The medicine* journey is organized by each energy center/chakra presenting its description, special characteristics, signs of imbalance, and a number of complementary healing options. Healing options include journaling and reflection exercises, meditation, opportunities to connect with the corresponding elements, and embodiment and holistic practices. By now, you may have a sense of the rhythm that works for you. Bringing energy healing into the mix can unearth what's been buried, so paying the sweetest attention to all of YOU is key. I think spending a good amount of time with each chakra allows for the realizations to come and for the medicine to take hold. You might decide to spend a few days or a week with each chakra or another pace altogether. There are a lot of options beloved, and you don't have to do it all; be practical, dear one. Healing be taking its tiiiiiime! In fact, it's written so that you can complete the journey intuitively with the guidance I'm offering this time and return in the future perhaps choosing a different combination of tools/practices. *body rites* really is here to meet you exactly where you are. Magical right?!

OK, so here's my flow recommendation, beloved |

FAMILIARIZE | Get to know the energy center. Take some time with the art; read through the descriptions and characteristics.

ASSESS | Notice what resonates or tells your story. Circle, highlight, make notes on the signs of imbalance that are familiar to your experience, as well as the aspects you feel are in harmony/personal strengths. This is not a pathologizing exercise. Remember, we are decolonizing, moving away from labeling what is human, signs of living, and reasonable responses to trauma as bad or wrong. Rather, this is an exercise of observation, introspection, and understanding. You are simply expanding your practice of NOTICING in ways that allow your intuition to reveal how your energy body has been impacted by past trauma—sexual trauma specifically.

REFLECT | Oh, beloved, you know I'm good for the journaling prompts. There are some gems up in here! Take your time—some are open-ended, others are sentence completion, and lastly there's space for creating your own positive affirmations as well. You're encouraged to write, draw, paint, imagine, collage, and tea or coffee stain all over these pages or a separate journal if preferred.

MEDITATE | There are meditation suggestions all over the medicine journey. Take your pick. I suggest making time for the chakra meditation created specifically for *the medicine journey* (instructions to follow). It may be most effective to return to this meditation for each energy center. Any additional meditation options are bonuses to be integrated as you discern.

PRACTICE | You might decide to make a plan or decide in the moment which healing practice you'd like to try. Keep in mind, some of the practices won't require anything but you and your body, while others will need supplies or preparation. My tip for the healing practices is to choose one from each of the three areas to start 1) element, 2) shapes, 3) holistic. Again, anything else you choose to add on, likely contingent on your pace and flow, is extra.

Other notes |

Lean on your opening and closing rituals from the 2nd journey as it feels right. Maybe they feel supportive with no change, but it'd also be OK to modify if that's where your intuition takes you. Using blessing herbs and sacred smokes before and after your practices are a wonderful option. You're invited to consult with your healing support team (e.g., shamans, guides, herbalists, energy healers, etc.) to determine any contraindications for known medical conditions, pregnancy, or other personal circumstances.

If you're being supported by a therapist or energy healer, you're encouraged to share what's coming up if it feels right as you work through.

SIGNS OF ENERGY RELEASE/SHIFTING |

When energy memories are stirred and coaxed to the surface by your healing intentions, old energy will naturally want to move out. The only thing it requires from you is allowance in the release. Signs of energy shifting or releasing are yawning, laughter, heat/temperature change, burping, coughing, tingling sensations, among others. Should you notice any of these signs, you might simply thank the energy for its lessons and thank your body for its release.

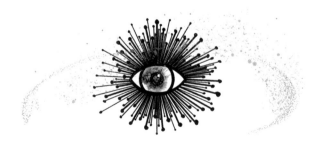

body rites

ENERGY CENTER MEDITATION INSTRUCTIONS |

Visualization is a practice, it takes time, remember it's OK if the mind wanders.

As you're ready with your inner eye, curiously, bring your attention to the energy center you'd like to focus on. As you visualize it, you might intuitively notice any colors, or textures that don't belong or seem out of place. As it feels right, see yourself clearing them out, perhaps sweeping, squeezing, plucking, or asking one of the elements for support. If you sense that the energy center is balanced and vibrant, you might simply offer gratitude. Notice any shifts or sensations of change. You're invited to complete the meditation by visiting your peaceful sacred space.*

---

* Energy center descriptions, aspects, qualities, and signs of disturbance are not exhaustive and draw from a collection of the texts previously mentioned.

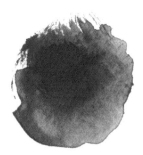

Root | survival and embodiment*

Color | red

Element | earth

Orisha | Shango

Affirmation | I have

Description | the most primal of the seven major energy centers as it is the foundation for our innate drives and basic needs, including survival, safety, security, and grounding.

Location | base of the spine

Sound | lam (lahm)

Planet | Saturn

Crystals | ruby, red jasper, garnet

Signs of disturbance |

    physical—sciatica, constipation, hemorrhoids, addiction, prone to illness

    psychological—fear, anxiety, rigidity, stubbornness, hyper-attachment, disorganized

JOURNALING PROMPTS + EXERCISES |

- Describe your connection to family.
- What's the current status of your basic needs, food, water, shelter, money? How do you feel about this?
- How would you describe your relationship with risk (adverse, healthy, addictive)?
- Which statement feels more true for you? *I rarely feel safe anywhere or with anyone. I sometimes feel like it's me against the world.* OR, *I feel safe a lot of the time, present in my body, and can relax into finding my way in the world.*

* FARM-P familiarize | assess | reflect (journal) | meditate | practice (elements, shapes, holistic)

body rites

- You're encouraged to complete the following statements as are truest for you.
  - I am safest when _____
  - When I hear the word abundance, I feel _____
  - My first instinct is to _____
  - My earliest memory of feeling safe is _____
  - My body _____
  - I am most grounded when _____
  - I connect with the earth by _____
- You're invited to create a positive affirmation for your root chakra practices by filling in the following: I have_____

GROUNDING + EARTHING PRACTICES |

- Plant or repot a plant
- Place your bare feet and/or walk on the grass or sand
- Lay down on the earth
- Hug a tree

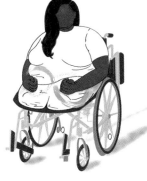

adhi mudra

SHAPES (OPTION TO PAIR WITH THE AFFIRMATION(S) YOU CREATED) |

- Adhi mudra
- Moforíbale
- Sitting on the earth/floor
- Inner child pose

HOLISTIC PRACTICES |

- Cook with root vegetables
- Eat/drink whole fruits and veggies on the red color spectrum
- Drink a cup of tea (recipe options to follow)

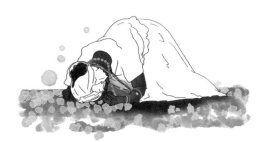

moforibale

REMEMBERING OUR ROOTS TEA |

- 1 part stinging nettles
- 1 part oat-straw

- ½ part burdock root
- ¼ part chicory root
- Optional: a pinch of cinnamon
- Blessed with a prayer/affirmation for remembering and recovering your roots
- Recommendation to drink 1 quart throughout the day for 21 days

Recommended as an herbal infusion to be taken as a tea. Please reference herbal preparations section for guidance and instructions. Remember this is your journey, follow your intuition in adding, omitting, and creating. For example, you might consider allowing this infusion to steep in the dark overnight and strain in the morning.

Tea notes |

Remember that the herbs are our allies and plant ancestors with living energy, intelligence, and memory. They are here to support. As you continue to build deeper intimacy with yourself, you're encouraged to be in reflection about your relationship with the plants you invite into your healing journey. A few suggestions for doing this are to develop a tea ritual for yourself, sit and smell the tea, take your time tasting it and observing what shows up mind, body, heart, and spirit. Here's some space to hold your notes.

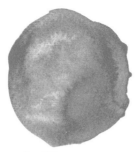

Sacral | sensuality, creativity, sense of self*

Color | orange

Element | water

Orisha | Yemoja

Affirmation | I feel . . .

Description | supports soul task of knowing and loving yourself, connecting with sensuality, emotions, sexuality, reproductivity, and creativity

Location | sacrum, lower abdomen, extends from pelvic bone up to the navel

Sound | vam (vahm)

Planet | moon

Crystals | moonstone, carnelian, amber

Signs of disturbance |

> physical—inflammation, gynecological problems, fertility challenges, low libido, menstrual irregularities, kidney issues

> psychological—insecure, indecisive, overindulgence, hyper-sensitive, lack of confidence, need for constant reassurance, sense of inadequacy, unworthiness

JOURNALING PROMPTS |

- When was the last time you created something?
- What's your relationship with pleasure?
- How do you know when you have compromised emotional boundaries? How do you know when you have healthy emotional boundaries?
- Which of the following statements feels more true? *Being sexually intimate with myself is intim-*

---

* FARM-P familiarize | assess | reflect (journal) | meditate | practice (elements, shapes, holistic)

body rites

idating, shameful, or uninteresting. OR, *when I am sexually intimate with myself, I feel open to exploring my body and experiencing pleasure.*

- You're encouraged to complete the following statements as are truest for you.
  - I am in touch with my emotions when _____
  - When I hear the word pleasure, my body _____
  - I am most sensual when _____
  - Going with the flow is _____
  - My sexuality is _____
  - I could honor my sensuality more by _____
  - I embody the element of water by _____
- You're invited to create a supportive affirmation for your sacral energy center practices by filling in the following: I feel _____

WATER + FLUIDITY PRACTICES |

- Spend time in or near a natural body of water
- Play in the rain
- Use watercolor to create a painting

SHAPES (OPTION TO PAIR WITH THE MANTRA(S) YOU CREATED) |

- Squat pose (Sanskrit name | malasana)
- Low crescent (Sanskrit name | anjaneyasana)
- Butterfly pose variations
- Hip nourishing and releasing shapes

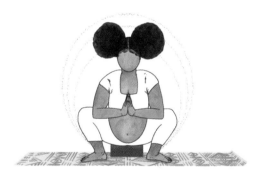

squat pose

HOLISTIC PRACTICES |

- Eat/drink whole fruits and veggies on the orange color spectrum
- Play music that inspires sensual movement
- Consider writing the personal story of your womb
- Bathe your crystals or special jewels in moonlight
- Take a dance class
- Create a pleasure plan (mind–body–heart–spirit is a trusted compass)
- Drink a cup of tea

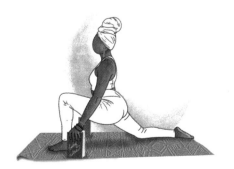

low crescent shape

SENSUALI-TEA |

- 1 part red raspberry leaf
- ½ part damiana
- ½ part rose petals
- ¼ hibiscus flower
- Optional: for extra nourishment and strength may include: 1 part red clover or corn silk
- Follow herbal tisane preparation
- Recommendation to drink warm during mooning cycle for beings who bleed
- Recommendations for testosterone-centered bodies: Add ½ part Saw Palmetto or Sarsaparilla
- Delicious when chilled in warmer months and/or combined with mineral water for bubbly enjoyment

CREATE & FLOW OIL |

- 1 part damiana
- ¼ part clove
- 1 vanilla bean
- ¼ part star anise
- ¼ part thyme
- Base oil (for example: grapeseed, avocado, sunflower, sesame, jojoba, olive oil)
- *Follow herbal oil preparation*
- If you're feeling adventurous, these ingredients work well as a space spray as well. You'll partner with the ingredients as though you are preparing an infusion, eliminating the oil. Steep overnight, strain, and add infusion (¾) to a dark spray bottle with (¼) witch hazel base, inviting a sensual decadent energy into your space.

Solar plexus | inner power*

Color | yellow

Element | fire

Orisha | Oshun

Affirmation | I do . . .

Description | concerned with the journey of personal power, fueling energy, assertiveness, and trust that we can live the life we want. This is where our personal will, self-determination, courage, and ability to set/maintain boundaries live.

Location | base of the sternum or between bottom ribs and the navel and governs more organs than any other energy center

Sound | ram (rahm)

Planet | mars

Crystals | tiger's eye, citrine, sunstone

Signs of disturbance |

> physical—digestive conditions/challenges, exhaustion, ulcers, gallstones, liver problems, adrenal imbalance

> psychological—quick-tempered, uncontrolled rage, aggression, impulsivity, numbness, lacking vitality, egotistical, self-centered, unhealthy relationship with food, powerlessness

JOURNALING PROMPTS |

- What words would you use to describe yourself (feel free to make a list, write a poem, recall lyrics to a song, etc.)?
- What are your personal strengths?

* FARM-P familiarize | assess | reflect (journal) | meditate | practice (elements, shapes, holistic)

- What's your relationship with anger? How do you know in your body when you are angry?

- Which of the following statements feels more true? *I often feel powerless, like there's not much I can do to change my circumstances for the better.* OR, *I am powerful beyond measure; I can shift my mindset and perspective in ways that help me to follow through with my intentions.*

- You're encouraged to complete the following statements as are truest for you.

  - I am most likely to follow through when _____

  - I am most powerful when _____

  - I struggle to hold my boundaries _____

  - I could honor my boundaries more by _____

  - I nurture my relationship with fire _____

- You're invited to create an encouraging affirmation for your solar plexus chakra practices by filling in the following: I do_____

FIRE PRACTICES |

- Light incense or a blessing herb at the beginning of your day

- Sun visualization meditation

- Have a private fire releasing ceremony creating a written list of things to release and burn it in a fire-safe container/cauldron

SHAPES (OPTION TO PAIR WITH THE MANTRA(S) YOU CREATED) |

- Warrior poses/sequences (Sanskrit name | virabhadrasana II)

- Core strengtheners

- Spinal twists

warrior II shape

HOLISTIC PRACTICES |

- Eat/drink whole fruits and veggies on the yellow color spectrum

- Cook with spice

- Explore your rage

- Joyful movement that brings warmth to your core

- Drink a cup of tea

INNER SUN TEA |

- 1 part lemon balm

- ½ part ginger root

- ¼ part fennel
- Optional: sweet orange peel (to amplify joyous power)
- *Follow herbal tisane preparation*

IN MY POWER OIL |

- Sweet orange peel
- Bitter orange peel
- Chamomile
- Cinnamon
- Orange blossom water
- Base oil of your choosing (e.g., avocado, sunflower, jojoba, olive oil)
- Optional: Black-eyed Susan flower essence
- Recommend infusing this oil for our inner sun (our solar plexus) with the medicine of the sun that lives in the sky by letting in daylight for a couple of hours
- *Follow herbal oil preparation*

body rites

Heart | love, compassion, alchemy*

Color | green or pink

Element | air

Orisha | Ogun

Affirmation | I love . . .

Description | commonly known as the bridge between the personal and spiritual energy centers and is concerned with the soul task of love, compassion, and alchemy

Location | situated behind the heart at the center of seven major energy centers

Sound | yam (yahm)

Planet | Venus

Crystals | emerald, rose quartz

Signs of disturbance |

> physical—hypertension, upper back/shoulder pain, immune compromised, nervous system disorders

> psychological—resentment, codependency, depression, over-identification with pain and suffering of others, minimizing logic, limited by past hurts

JOURNALING PROMPTS |

- What do you love about yourself?
- How do you show love to your body?
- How do you know when you have overextended yourself in love or compassion?
- What are some of the unhealthy patterns you repeat in romantic relationships?
- Which of the following statements feels more true? *I fall in love hard; I love people, places, and*

---

* FARM-P familiarize | assess | reflect (journal) | meditate | practice (elements, shapes, holistic)

body rites

things with all of me, sometimes to the point of losing myself. OR, *I have deep love for those I care about and am able to take care of myself and coexist with those close to me.*

- You're encouraged to complete the following statements as are truest for you.
  - I show compassion to myself by _____
  - Resentment is familiar to me, I feel it _____
  - My earliest memory of love _____
  - I offer compassion to others _____
  - When I feel unappreciated or unloved by others _____
  - I relate to the air element by _____
- You're invited to create an affirmation for your heart chakra practices by filling in the following: I love _____

AIR PRACTICES |

- Spend time outside
- Intentional breathing exercises
- Open the windows for fresh air

SHAPES (OPTION TO PAIR WITH THE AFFIRMATION(S) YOU CREATED) |

- Hands over the heart
- Crescent lunges with goal post arms
- Sphinx pose
- Heart openers
- Backbends

HOLISTIC PRACTICES |

- Eat/drink whole fruits and veggies on the green color spectrum
- Make a love themed playlist (self-love, love for others/world, healthy romantic love)
- Write a love note to yourself and put it somewhere you'll see daily
- Take yourself on a date or treat yourself to some extra self-care
- Take time to offer yourself loving touch
- Drink a cup of tea

HEART CENTERING TEA |

- 1 part rose
- 1 part tulsi
- ½ part hibiscus
- sweetener of your preference, maybe some sweetness from your lands or the lands you are on (e.g., honey, molasses, agave)
- Additional options:
  - Grief: ¼ part marigold (dried/fresh petals or flower essence)
  - Strengthening: ¼ part motherwort (dried/fresh or flower essence)
  - Protection: ¼ part elderflower (dried/fresh or flower essence)
- *Follow herbal tisane preparation*

TENDER LOVE CHEST OIL |

- ½ part hibiscus
- ½ part rose petals
- Recommended base: rose hip oil or other carrier oils are great options per your skin's constitution and accessibility
- *Follow herbal oil preparation*

Throat | expression, communication*

Color | blue

Element | ether

Orisha | Obatala

Affirmation | I speak, I hear

Description | known to hold information from the other energy centers and functions to support authentic expression, communication of truth, and ability to listen

Location | base of the throat

Sound | ham (haahm)

Planet | mercury

Crystals | turquoise, blue agate

Signs of disturbance |

> physical—sore throat, stiff neck, temporomandibular joint (TMJ), thyroid issues, ear, nose, and throat problems

> psychological—dishonesty, inability to verbalize, insensitivity, hyper-verbal

JOURNALING PROMPTS |

- When do you find it most challenging to communicate your truth?
- How would you describe your communication style?
- What would other people say about how you express yourself/communicate?
- When you dilute your truth or practice dishonesty, how does it feel in your body?
- Which of the following statements feels more true? *Sharing my truth with others is scary; I'm afraid that I will be judged, criticized, rejected, or worse, abandoned.* OR, *I am committed to*

---

* FARM-P familiarize | assess | reflect (journal) | meditate | practice (elements, shapes, holistic)

　　　　body rites

speaking my truth with intention and honor; I understand that in doing so I am also practicing authenticity, integrity, and self-respect.

- You're encouraged to complete the following statements as are truest for you.
  - I am most honest _____
  - I fear that in speaking my truth _____
  - I find it easiest to communicate with _____
  - I believe that most people say _____
  - I nourish my relationship with the ether by _____
- You're invited to create a positive affirmation for your throat chakra practices by filling in the following: I speak_____, I hear _____.

ETHER PRACTICES |

- Create or play with sound/instruments
- Say your name out loud first thing in the morning
- Explore connecting with ancestors or spirit guides
- Tell your story of transformation
- Sing your mantra

SHAPES (OPTION TO PAIR WITH THE AFFIRMATION(S) YOU CREATED) |

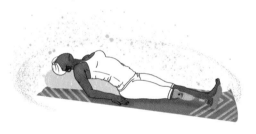

- Head/neck rolls
- Shoulder movements/openers
- Supported fish pose (Sanskrit name | matsyasana)
- Humming bee's breath

supported fish pose

HOLISTIC PRACTICES |

- Eat/drink whole fruits and veggies on the blue color spectrum, give special attention to how you present/arrange your food with beauty
- Hum or sing
- Say your prayers out loud
- Take some space
- Drink a cup of tea

SPEAK YOUR TRUTH TEA |

- 1 part chocolate mint leaves (option to substitute for spearmint or peppermint)
- ½ part chamomile
- ¼ part cloves
- Ginger root (to your taste)
- Recommendation to add warm coconut or oat milk and honey
- *Follow herbal tisane preparation*

BREATHE WITH EASE THROAT/CHEST OIL |

- 1 part spearmint or peppermint
- ½ part white pine
- ¼ part cedar or juniper
- Base oil of your choosing (coconut oil recommended)
- *Follow herbal oil preparation*

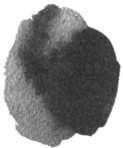

Third eye | insight, intuition, wisdom*

Color | Indigo, purple

Element | light

Orisha | Orunmila

Affirmation | I see . . .

Description | known as the center of inner vision and holds the ability to see into other realms, dimensions, and states of consciousness including ancestral memory and dreams. It is the wisdom we connect to through this energy center that supports our transcendence

Location | between the eyebrows

Sound | om or aum

Planet | Jupiter

Crystals | lapis lazuli, amethyst, sapphire

Signs of disturbance |

> physical—headaches, migraines, vision problems, sinusitis

> psychological—dismissiveness of personal spiritual experience, grief, confusion, mental fog, nightmares, abuse of your higher powers, skepticism

JOURNALING PROMPTS |

- How do you know when your intuition is speaking to you?
- What gets in the way of hearing your inner voice?
- How would you describe your dream practice, both sleeping and waking?
- Which of the following statements feels more true? *I'm not sure what the voice of my intuition sounds like or how it communicates with me; I don't dream very often and when I do, I tend to not*

---

* FARM-P familiarize | assess | reflect (journal) | meditate | practice (elements, shapes, holistic)

body rites

remember them. OR, *my inner voice is strong and I trust it; I dream most nights about different things and find reflecting about them is helpful.*

- You're encouraged to complete the following statements as are truest for you.

  - I often daydream about _____

  - When I ignore my intuition _____

  - I experience the most mental clarity when _____

  - I've noticed that I have more mental fog when _____

  - I fellowship with the light element by _____

- You're invited to create an encouraging affirmation for your third eye chakra practices by filling in the following: I see_____.

LIGHT PRACTICES |

- Day dream
- Keep a dream diary
- Spend time in the sun
- Candle flame meditation
- Meditate or sit at your altar between 4–6 a.m.

SHAPES (OPTION TO PAIR WITH THE AFFIRMATION(S) YOU CREATED) |

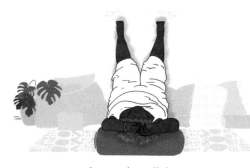

legs up the wall shape

- Meditation in a shape of your choice that allows the spine to be long
- Legs up the wall shape
- Inversions
- Alternate nostril breathing (instructions to follow)

HOLISTIC PRACTICES |

- Create a vision board
- Bathe your water or tea in the sun
- Journey with cannabis, ayahuasca, iboga, or peyote**
- Drink a cup of tea

**advised to seek the guidance of a trusted elder/healer and with respect to the source/native lands of the plant ancestors*

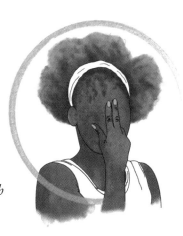

alternate nostril breathing mudra

ALTERNATE NOSTRIL BREATHING (SANSKRIT NAME | NADI SHODHANA)

- *Option 1*
  - Take a full in breath through the nose and out breath through the mouth as you're ready. Connect with a flow of inhalations/exhalations through the nose.
  - Allow the eyes to make a choice.
  - If you're able, gently place the right index and middle finger to the third eye. Press the right thumb to the right nostril, and inhale through the left nostril. Press the left nostril closed with the right ring finger, releasing the thumb to exhale out the right nostril. Inhale right nostril, apply thumb to exhale left nostril.
  - Repeat inhalation/exhalation, alternating breath flow through left and right nostrils. You're invited to breath this way for 7–11 cycles, finishing with an exhale out of the left nostril.
  - When you're ready release the mudra. You're encouraged to observe any sensations in the body, noticing any shifts.
- *Option 2*
  - Another option is to not use the mudra and to concentrate on breathing through one nostril at a time following the same flow described above.

IN MY VISIONS TEA |

- 1 part tulsi
- ½ part mugwort
- ¼ part blue lotus
- Optional: ¼ part cannabis leaves
- *Follow herbal tisane preparation*

ILLUMINATION SPRAY |

- ½ part lavender
- ½ part rosemary
- ½ lemon peel
- Base: witch hazel or rubbing alcohol
- *Follow herbal tisane preparation* if you are using fresh herbs, strain, and combine ½ part herbal water, ½ part base of choice, pouring into a dark amber or glass spray bottle. Alternatively, you might use herbal essential oils when fresh herbs are not accessible or preferred. Recommendations to spray over the head for clarity and connection, in your physical space, on the hair after wash day, or as a part of beginning/end of day rituals.

crown | divine connection, liberation*

Color | white, gold, violet

Element | pure spirit

Orisha | Ori

Affirmation | I know . . .

Description | our sacred place of divine connection and freedom, this energy center helps us to realize, fulfill, and experience bliss through spiritual practice

Location | crown of the head

Sound | silence

Planet | Sun, Uranus

Crystals | clear quartz, selenite

Signs of disturbance |

>   physical—chronic fatigue, hyper-sensitivity to light, sound, or environment

>   psychological—worry, depression, feeling of emptiness, fragmented

JOURNALING PROMPTS |

- What are your signs of healing? How are you different since beginning the medicine journey?
- Describe your relationship with the "divine" and spirit. What's shifted or new?
- What are your grateful for?
- Which of the following statements feels more true? *I don't know how to connect to my divinity, God, or spirit. I am restless, worry all the time, and feel like a stranger in my body.* OR, *I am divine. I am at peace. I am supported. I am protected. I know what being at home in my body feels like.*

* FARM-P familiarize | assess | reflect (journal) | meditate | practice (elements, shapes, holistic)

- You're encouraged to complete the following statements as are truest for you.
  - My spirit is _____
  - My path to liberation _____
  - When obstacles present themselves, I can _____
  - I am worthy of _____
  - These things I know for sure _____
  - I cultivate my relationship with spirit by _____
- You're invited to create a supportive affirmation for your crown chakra practices by filling in the following: I know_____.

SPIRIT PRACTICES |

- Rest and quality sleep
- Prayer and altar work
- Ritual
- Spiritual baths
- Give thanks

SHAPES (OPTION TO PAIR WITH THE AFFIRMATION(S) YOU CREATED) |

- Meditation in silence, holding your head if it feels right
- At home in your body

HOLISTIC PRACTICES |

- Foot massages and reflexology
- Unplug/go off the grid
- Yoga Nidra
- Be mindful of sugar intake/processed foods
- Drink a cup of tea

COOL CROWN TEA |

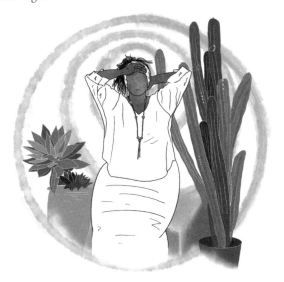

hands holding head shape

- 1 part Gotu kola
- ¼ part mint leaves
- Ginger root (to your taste)
- Option to drink cool and add fresh squeezed lemon and basil ice cubes
- *Follow herbal tisane preparation*

CROWN BLESSING BATH |

- ½ part rosemary
- 1 bay leaf
- 1–2 handfuls of purple and/or white flower petals
- ¼ part lavender
- Leaves from a tree in your region (e.g., white pine, cedar, juniper, pinion)
- Full pinch of natural salts (e.g., celtic, pink Himalayan, sea salts)
- 1–2 cups of coconut milk
- For extra sweetness and gentleness: calendula and/or rose water
- *Follow herbal bath preparation. Allow to cool before use.*
- Recommendation is to shower or bathe as you would normally. Turn off the water and choose a shape of reverence, perhaps kneeling in the tub if you are able, pouring the bath from your bowl onto your head and over your body. Allow your body to air dry and consider wrapping the head with a white piece of material or T-shirt.

body rites

4th Journey | *spirit & the ancestors*

May we have the awareness and clarity to look back into the existence of loving and nurturing ancestors. May we allow our stories to start in a time of togetherness and the essence of joy. Although some of our ancestors who are close to us may have been the very reason for some of the trauma we carry, we will claim a newness of unhealthy cycles being broken.

May we understand that what lies within our DNA is that of greatness, and although there are traces of struggle, there is a genesis of the power to heal and love purely.

What lies within me is the power to heal. I choose to learn new ways of being. I am seeking the knowledge of making myself complete mentally, emotionally, and spiritually. I call on those who have come before me to ignite the flame of my ancestors, so I may move in the grace and strength of the hundreds that have come before, those who lift me to new realms on a daily basis.

I am capable. I love myself enough to gently apply all of the tools that have been divinely placed in front of me. I will be gentle with myself because I deserve to be cared for. This journey may not be easy but I recognize today that I am worthy of telling my story from a gaze of deep self-knowing rooted in awareness. I am capable of shaping my story in a new way and in doing so I will rise to new heights fueled by love and sweetness. I am ready for a new me.

—prayer offered by Iya Fayomi Osundoyin Egbeyemi

Beloved, your healing is so powerful, it reaches forward and backward at the same time. When you hold space for yourself, you touch the past and change the future. I am so moved by you and your commitment to healing. Welcome to the fourth and final journey of the *body rites* ceremony. It is at once a prayer of gratitude, a numinous inquiry, and an invitation to deepen relationships with your ancestors as a source of support in healing yourself and intergenerational trauma. This rite beckons you to consider how the wounds of your ancestors are carried in your body, DNA, and ways of being. You'll be invited to pace yourself through a series of moments and rituals rooted in African spirituality intended to evoke curiosity, ancestral connection, and intergenerational healing. Take your time.

INTERGENERATIONAL TRAUMA |

Intergenerational trauma, also sometimes referred to as ancestral or historical trauma, refers to the ways in which our bloodlines' traumas live on in our bodies, in relationship dynamics/ patterns, and our belief systems. Trauma stored in the body has been proven to exist on a cellular level and in our DNA. We literally carry the stories of our ancestors and elders in our bodies and nervous systems. The crystallization of these stories, particularly the traumatic aspects, can show up in uncanny ways. For instance, in remembering the metaphysical and energetic aspects of trauma, fibroids in the maternal line could indicate history of sexual trauma. I think of fibroids (not in all cases) as tumors of violation or intrusion, often sexual in nature. This can be said of endometriosis and other reproductive issues as well. That the energy of sexual trauma takes up space, festers, and grows uninvited in the body. Mama Koko Zauditu Selassie, Lucumi priestess and elder star of *In Our Mothers' Gardens*, says "the wombs are wounded." Similarly, high blood pressure could be rooted in history of chronic stress in the bloodline. Generations of Black bodies contracting in response to abuse, surviving against the odds, and harboring the holistic assaults of white supremacy can certainly create a pressurized bodily ecosystem—and inevitably intergenerational epidemics amongst people of African ancestry.

It goes deeper, beloved. I mentioned that we carry our ancestors with us in our DNA. I'd like to geek out with you for a minute in the science of it all. Did you know that females in utero carry all their eggs? So, this means, when our great-grandmother was pregnant with our grandmother, our grandmother was housing the egg of what would become our mother . . . and so on. Isn't that powerful, that for a moment in time there is a sharing of the same body or concentric bodies? And so, doesn't it make sense, that their stories, lived experiences, and trauma are encoded in our DNA? This is a sacred position. We know the things that we ourselves do not have the life experience for, but also host painful wounds in our bodies. This is one of the reasons there might be themed struggles and ways of being within the family lineage.

There's some work to do here. I invite you into compassionate observation of the wounds that thrive in your bloodline, those that show up in various forms across the family trees, and those that drain and undermine the vitality of you and your kindred. This often shows up as unhealthy patterns passed down from generation to generation, as substance dependence/

abuse, incest/sexual trauma, self-sabotage, toxic intimate relationships, limiting parenting skills, codependency, and distorted belief systems to name a few. Collectively, we have become really creative in matters of coping and surviving. Actually, while we are here, I'd like to share some thoughts about codependency.

The term codependency can elicit feelings of shame or embarrassment due to stigma. I like to dispel that because I believe codependency has beginnings as a survival skill/tool, particularly for enslaved Africans and subsequently passed down to their descendants. Our ancestors were expected and forced to caretake for their abusers in various forms, in order to survive. Thinking about that as descendants of enslaved Africans makes the connection for us. Codependency can be viewed as a byproduct of enslavement, perhaps even a contemporary symptom of post traumatic slave syndrome (DeGruy, 2017). I am specifically speaking to the caretaking aspects of codependency. Melody Beattie states "that the behaviors associated with codependency are behaviors that saved our lives when we didn't know what else to do" and that "there are times we do too much, care too much, feel too little, or overly engage" (Beattie, 2009, p. 10). I define codependency as a compromised ability to see ourselves independent of the identities, needs, and expectations of others. It becomes a way of being that centers the experience of others, necessitating incremental or large actions of self-abandonment and is influenced by emotional interest in pleasing others.

From the trauma lens, I might offer that codependency is kindred to the "tend and befriend" trauma response we explored in a previous journey. That we inherited through DNA and intergenerational patterns this way of relating to others. The ways in which we make choices, appease others, people please, take care of, or nurture others at the expense of ourselves, our truths, and in some cases as a means of survival. So, during conflict in the context of an abusive, manipulative, violent relationship, or unhealthy power dynamic, one might abandon or dilute their truth to deescalate the situation. This might look like over-assuming responsibility, ignoring your intuition, dismissing the facts, moving toward the threat, or compromising personal boundaries to name several examples.

As you're reading, you may be noticing what wants to come to the surface to be recognized. Some of the intergenerational wounds and patterns may be easy to identify, while others require you to delve deeply. As you're reflecting on the intergenerational wounds or harmful patterns that show up in your family lineages, you might consider inclinations to substance abuse, toxic communication styles, incest, parental abandonment, and emotional neglect as examples.

You are not beholden to the way it's been for so long. The cycle can end with you.

You're invited to identify 3–5 intergenerational wounds within your family lines and/or cultures.

How might these intergenerational wounds/patterns have been tools of survival at one time?

Explore how you might commit to healing and transcending these wounds in your own life and body.

What will it take to break the cycle(s)? Which of these things are within your control?

body rites

How would things need to change or be different?

How would YOU need to change or move differently?

You're invited to create a vision statement for your family bloodline(s) moving forward.

What are the values you'd like your family to be rooted in moving forward?

If it feels right, you might use the space on the next page to create or collage a vision board inspired by your responses.

When we commit to our healing, we break and end cycles.
And we become liaisons for the healing of our ancestors and future generations.

When we hold space for ourselves that asserts the existence of intergenerational trauma, we cultivate an environment to heal on a cellular level. The embodiment practices and holistic tools you have been exploring throughout the *body rites* ceremony, intimately inform healing that can change the expression of your genes so that the old painful stuff doesn't get passed on through the body. This is the magic of epigenetics.

There's something about how my people survived, became themselves, how they equipped generations that followed, for better or for worse, that makes me burst with compassion and respect. They did the best they could with what they had. And I feel so empowered in knowing that some of what they had, their best aspects, their wisdom, courage, and power, their ability to alchemize, I also carry in my being. As do you, beloved.

What are the themed strengths evident in your bloodlines and/or family lineages? These are the undeniable best aspects of your family members that show themselves over and over across generations. For example, I come from women who are infinitely creative and are not afraid to love.

What do you and yours have in common?

By now, dear one, you are likely in a steeping relationship with your intuition. In previous *body rites* journeys, you were encouraged to notice the spiritual impact of sexual trauma—perhaps as an injury to your intuition, sense of purpose, or connection to a higher power. And you were called into the opportunity and urgency of repairing relationship with intuition as something to reclaim. In the fourth and final *body rites* journey, you're being invited to explore the rich union between your intuition and your ancestors.

That longing you are holding—the craving of closeness you feel deep down—so many of us are feeling it. The heightened sensitivity, the secret curiosity, and research you are indulging in about the traditions you've heard of, the vivid dreams you seem to be having, the palpable knowing that you are not alone. It is in the recognition of these sensations that they become a a less surreal experience. Consequentially, perhaps we become more attuned to the subtleties of spirit. When we sink into our bodies and notice spiritual sensations and presence, we fortify the communication and the channel between us and our ancestors—spirit. Our intuition is a vessel for our higher self, ancestors, and spiritual guides to speak to us. In being able to sense into our intuition with clarity and being able to differentiate it from the sensations of our traumas misleading us, we access an expanded consciousness in our bodies and spirits. What if when your ancestors speak to you through your intuition, they are creating a path that inspires remembrance, reclamation, and space to explore?

Where in your body do you feel the longing for connection with your beloved ancestors?

You're encouraged to search yourself for this place, bringing your attention or hands there if it feels right and you are able. You might take a few breaths in acknowledgement.

> *This is the space in my body where the longing lives.*
> *Where I long to connect with my ancestors.*
> *To know them, to sit with them,*
> *to hear them, to feel them.*
> *In time.*
> *Àṣẹ.*

And if by chance you are noticing resistance—and you might—now and beyond, I invite you to center in your curiosity and explore what's coming up. You may even take a moment to notice how resistance is showing up in your body as sensations, constriction, changes in your breath . . .

> *"Somehow, I knew that there was much more going on*
> *than was apparent on the surface.*

My existence and that of the things going on around me caused me to question everything, always looking for the deeper meanings."

—Iya Luisah Teish on Growing up Tipsy (Jambalaya, p. 3)

HERE ARE SOME QUESTIONS THAT MAY BE HELPFUL TO EXPLORE |

Am I experiencing fear?

If so, where did this fear come from?

Is it mine or was it left with me?

Who does this fear protect?

Am I afraid of remembering what has been forgotten? If so, why?

Perhaps you are making connections to family, religious beliefs, the wounds of White supremacy, oppression, and genocide. It's amazing to consider what we will forget, if it's a circumstance of life or death. You are not alone in what may be bubbling up. There's a long violent history of our ancestral lineages and wisdoms being demonized and weaponized. These agendas have been carried forward in organized religion and churches, indoctrinating our communities, conditioning fear and shame in relationship to our ancient traditions. This is one of the many manifestations of spiritual or church traumas. Some of the degenerative conditioning we've been victimized by, has resulted in externalizing our intuitive process, relinquishing our trust to someone ordained to facilitate connection with a higher power(s) and ancestors.

Does any of this sound familiar?

Let the dead rest.

Worshipping ancestors is a sin.

Ancestor veneration is witchcraft.

These are lies.

Through your intuition/inner knowing, you have a direct path to your spiritual family. Am I telling your story again, beloved? You've likely heard some version of one or all of these sayings. How has this affected your connections or pursuit of relationships with your ancestors?

When you were a younger self, did you experience special senses/connections you seemed to lose as you got older?

You might be noticing some tension between what you've been taught and what you'd like to explore. It is yours to discover, and yours to remember. Would it be OK to give yourself permission to acknowledge the questions coming up as an opening. Or maybe you are feeling fully charged to move in closer, maybe this all feels natural and nostalgic in some way. Wherever you are is just right.

I invite you to take a breath in, exhale a breath out, maybe noticing any sensations that are arising. If it feels right, maybe returning to connection with that place in your body where the longing lives. You know more than you know, beloved.

What questions do you have about ancestral reverence?

You may already have spiritual practices that support being in regular intimate communication and relationship with your ancestors. Maybe you have questions you'd like to ask them directly on the topics of healing. You're invited to make notes in the space provided on the following page.

body rites

This might be just enough for now. You're supported in honoring where you are. If you'd like to continue exploring ancestral reverence as a healing path, I'll be offering some ritual suggestions later in the journey. In the meantime, I've listed a few practices/prompts to explore and make your own.

WAYS TO BE IN COMMUNITY WITH YOUR ANCESTORS |

Consider how you might already be in conversation and community with them. In your daily movements, the heirlooms you cherish, the placement of photos of your ancestors in your spaces, the foods you love that feed your soul, the musical totems that stir you.

You might consider identifying 3–4 ancestors you respect, a quality that you revere for each, and one part of their legacy you remember.

What are the stories you most often tell about your ancestors?

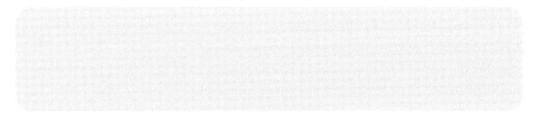

Where are the places you visit/frequent that you feel their presence at its strongest?

I've offered in moments throughout the *body rites* ceremony that I draw from a wealth of sources, tangible and intangible. My work and personal practices are in part anchored in West African spirituality, specifically the Yoruba traditions of Ifá. There's so much to share about this, that is beyond the scope of this book, and with respect to the many traditions, religions, and wisdoms we collectively hold as sacred. My intention is not to inject a spiritual philosophy, enforce a belief system, or to suggest any singular religious trajectory. This rite is an invitation and continuation of efforts to indigenize individual, collective, and ancestral healing in partnership with curiosity, remembrance, and discovery in the spiritual body. As always, take what you need and leave the rest here.

As a little one, raised by the women in my family—some of whom were religious and others who were religious adjacent—I had the reputation of being "too smart for my own good." I asked the questions that no one ever seemed to have the answers for, or perhaps the forbidden questions whose answers were buried underneath fear, indoctrination, repression, genocide, and epistemicide. In her sweet voice and bright narrow eyes, little Shena would ask "What did we believe in before we were brought over here on boats?" I was drawn to the fragile, antique things I wasn't supposed to touch. I felt things in the rooms and corners of houses no one else seemed to notice; I had sweet dream-visits from folk I had never met but somehow knew were family. I would get lost in a trance from dancing. I could sometimes feel what was coming before it happened. I knew things that I had not lived. I *know* things that I have not lived.

You might be able to imagine how it felt in my seeking and curiosity to discover some of the answers to my questions as an adult. This has been one of the most profound and empowering aspects of my healing journey. Allowing the questions and curiosity to alchemize the fear, to challenge the conditioning, and to create an opening for remembrance and reclamation. These are just a few of the things that have happened. The spiritual simmering turned into a boiling, a cauldron, and an ongoing unfolding.

The landscape for exploring African spiritual practices and ancestral veneration/reverence is vast, and again much larger than what I can squeeze into the remaining pages of our *body rites*. I'd like to offer opportunities for play and exploration of healing in the elements and finally a series of rituals. I'm excited for your moments.

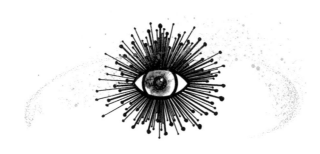

body rites

Thank you to the elements for their brilliance
For being everywhere and anywhere

To the wind
May we be carried gently, may we BE wildly in it

To the fire
May it burn away the outgrown

In water
May we not be afraid to face the current, to resist it
May we be soft enough to go forward with it

On earth
May we stand on it
without breaking it

We are elemental people. We come from people with wholesome, rich, illustrious relationships with the elements. People who commune and respect the elements as teachers, spirits, time capsules, and proverb muses. In presencing ourselves with various animations of nature, in being humble students, observers, and intimate partners with the elements we can become more dynamic versions of ourselves. It is no coincidence that people proclaim a need to spend more time outside when stressed, that they find it easier to breathe when in close proximity to the ocean, or that a rain storm feels cleansing. In African spiritual traditions across the diaspora, there is an intimate relationship between nature elements and Orisha. As our enslaved ancestors were deposited in various parts of the world, they did what we do—they got creative. They held on tight to spiritual traditions, masked them with songs and European idols, fought literal and spiritual wars with them, protected them, and evolved them to partner with their fortitude to survive past their flesh. In many corners of the diaspora, we know these traditions as Ifá, Lucumí, Santería, and Voudon. Intimate relationship between the elements and Orisha prevail and pulse through all of the respective iterations of these African religions.

I invite you into a moment of meditation and reflection, inspired by *Indigenous Tools for Living (ITFL)*, created by Shirley Turcotte. As you're ready, pause and consider, if you were a piece of nature right now, what would you be? Gently allowing yourself to feel the sensations of becoming and being this piece of nature. You're invited to stay here as long as you'd like, perhaps for 10–20 breath cycles.

You're invited to journal in the space below, considering what your felt experience as a piece of nature came to show you. What medicine did it bring?

How do you hold spirituality in your body? Does it show up as earth, water, fire, wind, or some other expression?

ORISHA |

The Orisha, once human, were appointed by Olodumare (creator) and elevated to deities. There are numerous Orisha, however, there are seven primary divine beings reverenced and represented across the diasporic spectrum of African traditional religions (with name variations/pronunciations depending on language/specific tradition). Obatala, Esu-Elegba, Yemoja, Oshun, Ogun, Sango, and Oya, in their respective ways of being, embody aspects of nature, life essence, and aspirational qualities/characteristics. As deified beings, they come to help us develop good character in our human experience, to aid in our spiritual development, and to bolster the connection between our consciousness and behavior. The Orisha are multifaceted and beautifully complex in their attributes, physical correspondences, and elemental, energetic, and cosmic aspects. It is through intimate relationship, practice, and experience that we are able to embody and manifest within ourselves the best in each of them, and ultimately our own divine expressions of God.

What are you noticing, beloved?

Are there signs of resistance or discomfort?

Is there anything in nature that can hold this for you?

Where are you noticing sensations of resonance and curiosity in your body?

You're invited to explore the following charts* adapted from various sources on African and Yoruba spiritual wisdoms. As you explore, you might notice the attributes you feel most aligned with, those you experience challenges or imbalance in, areas in the body you feel strong or perhaps where you struggle with ailments/dis-ease; allowing any meaning or intuitive message to crystallize.

Orisha	Attributes	Nature Element	Physical Correspondence
Obatala	Elder of the Orisha | wisdom, purity, peacemaker	Mountains, woods	Brain, bones, white fluids of the body
Esu-Elegba	Messenger of the Orisha and guardian of the crossroads | Keeper of Àṣẹ, gate-keeper/opener of the way, trickster	Crossroads, gateways	Sympathetic nervous system, para-sympathetic nervous system
Yemoja	The great mother | nurturer, cleansing, sexuality	Salt water oceans/ lakes	Womb, liver, breasts, buttocks
Oshun	Spirit of the river | love, sensuality, beauty, fertility, equality	Fresh water rivers/ lakes	Circulatory system, digestive organs, elimination system, pubic area (female)
Ogun	Spirit of Iron | Path clearer, truth, protection, war, justice	Woods/forests, forges	Heart, kidney, and adrenal glands, tendons
Oya	Spirit of the wind | death, rebirth, transformation/ change	Cemetery, wind, storms, thunder	Lungs, bronchial passages, mucous membranes
Sango	Spirit of lightning | strength, cour-age, vigor, passion, virility	Base of trees, light-ning, fire	Reproductive sys-tem (male), bone marrow, life force or chi

*chart adapted from information in various resources, including Karade, 1994, p. 30; Teish, 1985, Afedefeyo, 2017. Readers should note this chart is not exhaustive. You are encouraged to delve into available resources for a more comprehensive review of Orisha and ATRs.

body rites

You're invited to continue exploring intimate connection with your ancestors in support of your healing. Maybe there are discoveries or things you'd like to integrate from your *body rites* journey. I've offered some guidance and suggested rituals to make your own and return to as often as it feels right.

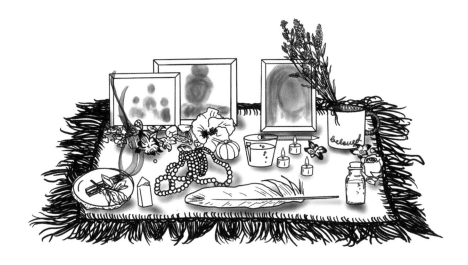

ALTAR BUILDING |

You might explore creating an ancestral altar if you haven't already. Follow your intuition in determining the details—location and what to include. Draping the altar with a white cloth and decorating with a white candle, glass of water, maybe a small plant, and any photos or special heirlooms is a beautiful beginning.

You're invited to explore the following rituals for *ancestral support in your healing, ancestral healing, and for your future.*

Ritual for ancestors supporting your healing

This ritual offers an opportunity to tap into the intergenerational and vicarious aspects of ancestral healing. Remembering that just as we carry their stories and wounds with us, we also hold within us the best in each of them.

Where do you feel your ancestors' strengths, transcendent wisdoms, joy, sovereignty, love, pride in your body?

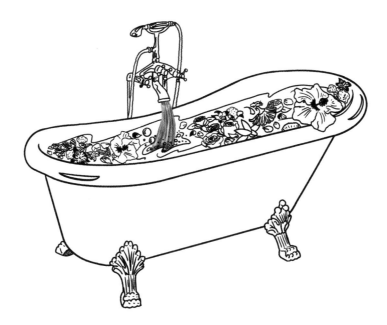

You might consider making an offering to your altar by cooking a meal. What are the foods that are special to your family and culture? You might serve the meal on a white plate, placing it on the altar for no more than three days.

I shared an herbal bath recipe with you in the third body rite, divined to bring coolness to the head (Ori) and to assist the connection with your intuition and spiritual support. The fourth rite spiritual bath invites you to call upon your elevated ancestors and spiritual squad to support your healing. I've included those instructions below.

Option 1 | Combine 4 cups of coconut milk, ¼ cup of honey, and sliced oranges in a bowl. As you are preparing your spiritual bath, you're invited to say a clear prayer of how you would like spirit and your beloved ancestors to support you. Remember your words are powerful incantations. Pray fervently for what you need and so deserve. You might consider some of the persistent themes you've noticed throughout your journey. For example, challenges with self-love, worthiness, or self-sabotage. Run a full bath and pour the bowl of spiritual ingredients into the water. I'd also encourage you to consider adding fresh flowers to your bath. As you're ready, you're encouraged to immerse your whole body in the bath, if you are able, while reflecting on your prayers: what you're calling in, what you're releasing, and what you need in support. When it feels right, let the water drain out of the tub, air dry, and wrap your body with a white sheet, towel, or cloth.

If accessing a bathtub is not possible or comfortable, you can modify for a shower. While in your shower, you might decide to stand or choose a shape of reverence, perhaps kneeling if you are able, pouring the bath from your bowl onto your head and over your body. Allow your body to air dry and consider wrapping the head with a white piece of material or T-shirt.

You're invited to journal freely in the following space, noticing what comes up, or how you feel before, during, and after your bath.

Ritual for ancestral healing

Where do the wounds of your ancestors live in your body? You might focus on specific individuals or groups (e.g., maternal lineage) related by a particular identity, time, or shared experience (e.g., sexual trauma) as an option; naming/acknowledging it so that it can be transformed.

Is there anything from your ancestors' experiences/stories that could be helpful to you now? You might explore one being at a time or address the collective if it feels right, perhaps remembering the wounded themes you identified in previous reflections.

Is there an Orisha or element of nature you'd like to ask for support in this ritual?

You're invited to make note of any symbolism/images, sensations, or urges that come up.

This next ritual leans into nature and water for support in healing ancestral/intergenerational wounds. It may require some planning and patience to see it through. Know that your timing is divine. When it feels right, you're encouraged to take a journey to a body of water, if possible wearing all white. When you arrive, greet the water, observe its qualities, feel its first touch. Take your time and see if you might be able to see yourself in its reflection, to see the reflection of those in your bloodline. When it feels right, you're invited to enter the water, name the wounds, and put them into the water with your words. Wash yourself with the water, for you and for them. As you're ready, immerse yourself in the water completely. Once may be enough—or you might feel called to repeat any of these steps multiple times. When you're ready, you might offer gratitude to the body of water for its support. Exit the water looking forward and moving away from all that you are leaving behind.

Ritual for ancestors supporting your future/destiny

They have your back and want to support your dreams. You're invited to take some time to search yourself and imagine your future.

How do you want to be?

What do you imagine for your destiny? Is there anything worth reimagining?

What can you draw from in your relationship/connection with your ancestors in support of your destiny?

You're encouraged to write a letter to your ancestors, on a separate sheet of paper, naming what you want for yourself/your life and to request their support. Be specific, beloved. Help them to see, feel, smell, taste, and touch it as you do. You might partner with an element and/or Orisha, as it feels right. You're invited to smear your letter with the sacred resins of frankincense and myrrh. When it feels right, read the letter aloud and burn it in a fire-safe cauldron or pit. If working with fire is not aligned, you might consider digging a hole in soil to plant it in the earth.

Know that these rituals are here for you as much as you'd like to lean on them for support. Make them your own and change them as you are changing. As we move toward closure, I'd like to share a poem given to me by the ancestors during one of my first *healing on the mat* workshop cycles. The survivor–participants were halfway through the series and had begun to notice what seemed like serendipitous connections between them, what seemed like coincidental life moments, a new rawness and sensitivity within, and revelations that some of their ways of BEING were in tandem with spirit. It was a magnificent and powerful opening.

A MESSAGE FROM THE ANCESTORS FOR OUR COLLECTIVE |

we are here for you.

we are proud of you.

you are doing the thing we couldn't do.

and we respect you.

let fear not corrupt your healing.

you are worthy to be fearless in your body.

it is yours after all.

can you BE in it, like you mean it?

BE in it like you mean it, baby.

and know that we are here.

we mean it.

we love you.

àṣẹ.

CLOSURE |

Oh beloved, it's been such a pleasure to call you that in our time together. Thank you for being here, for choosing to heal. I am immensely proud *with* you; however, you have chosen to journey through these body rites. Closure is here.

What does that mean to you? Drawing upon all that you have gathered along the way, how would you like to end this ceremony?

You're invited to take some time to consider what feels right.

You're encouraged to return to any healing intentions, love notes, poems, or letters you wrote in previous body rites. Noticing what has changed, what's been rearranged, and what remains since you began the *body rites* healing ceremony.

What is it like to be you—in mind, body, heart, and spirit?

How has your relationship with your body changed?

When healing times get tough, what do you need to remember?

What's next on your healing journey?

As always, there is space below to reflect and to capture the moments.

body rites

May the healing continue.
May it be a place you return to.
A nostalgia your body longs for.
A space you choose to be
For however long it takes.

May the healing continue, beloved. Know that you can return to these body rites as often as you need to. I've offered a few suggestions for allowing all that's within these pages—all the tools you have collected—to support you in healing that is enduring and intuitive. As always, there is space to write in your own ideas and intentions as well.

- Review your notes.
- Share your observations and insights with your therapist.
- Make a list of your favorite tools, shapes, and rituals for quick reference when you need them most.
- Consider revisiting activities/sections of the book as it feels right, make them your own.
- Work what you've learned into your daily rhythm.

Beloved, as I've written these poems, strung these body rites together, channeled these words, touched rivers, sat by my altars and in my body, I have held you so close. I've imagined you holding this book, tears and tea stains on its pages, healing discussions lifting up out of it, and that in every moment you seep into another space inside your body. That in turning these pages and shifting shapes, your intuition becomes the loudest part of you, that your ancestors move in to touch and be touched by the alchemy you have created in choosing to reclaim your body sovereignty. I've become overwhelmed by envisioning all of us, the potent and palpable healing between us, among us, and beyond us because we chose ourselves. Because we listened to our bodies and perhaps felt like it might feel right to live inside them, *where we belong*.

body rites

epilogue |

This epilogue is written for anyone that holds space for Black survivors of sexual trauma: therapists, healing-practitioners, helping professionals, biological and chosen family members, besties, lovers, and partners. *You are the healing companions.* This is an invitation to collectively shift the standards of holding space in ways that celebrate the power, intuition, and bottomless healing capacity of Black survivors. It is an invitation to reckon with the harmful aspects and limitations of traditional mental healthcare and to reimagine care that tends to the whole being.

This is a precious space of holding.

I imagine that you are here because you love someone that has been hurt. That you have held someone trying to move back in or find home in a Black body that someone else felt entitled to. That you've witnessed the size of their emotional waves and wondered how they manage to keep swimming. That you've seen them wander outside of themselves, noticed moments of vacancy in their eyes, felt them tremble, go numb, or lose their way. You've watched their heart break or perhaps, to your naked eye, nothing seemed to change at all. Maybe you've heard their secrets and stories, listened closely as they pulled fragmented memories together to paint a picture. You've seen how they blame and doubt themselves about what happened, all the while their bodies are screaming emissions of all the details their minds can't recall.

You've likely also been touched by their glory, moved by their creativity, comforted by their warmth, and inspired by their tenacity.

Maybe you are also *them*—you've been hurt, traversing both spaces—survivor and space holder or healing companion.

I am so deeply grateful that you are here. That you are choosing to expand your embrace, anchor into humility, and coat the space you hold for survivors in curiosity. I'm biased—I believe that holding space for Black survivors of sexual trauma is one of the most sacred and intimately nuanced positions one can be in. I hope that in picking up this book you can remember what it's like to hold something you cherish.

> *May survivors know in their bodies that we*
> *believe them, we cherish them, we see them,*
> *and that we are committed to holding*
> *precious space for their embodied return . . .*
> *it is the absolute least we can do.*

This is not an instructional chapter that will tell you how to heal Black survivors. It is not a prescription pad of quick fixes or escape routes. It is not an academic recapitulation of theories or a manual for people wanting to become experts in sexual trauma work. It is certainly not written by a master with all the tools and rules in healing.

It is an opening, a relationship, and a responsibility.

If you're noticing sensations of disappointment, I invite you to ask yourself why.

Oftentimes, we read books with the intention of telling others about themselves or how to figure out their stuff. We look for language or nomenclature to categorize and to pathologize. These intentions are not inextricable from alienation. Sure, it's easier to see what's wrong or needs saving about someone else, and likely more challenging to see ourselves and the role we play implicitly and explicitly. Being a healing companion of *body rites* is a parallel process. It is an opportunity to engage in self inquiry, to explore embodiment, and perhaps even offer a salve to some of your own wounds. I believe the most impactful support a person or community can receive comes from people who persist in commitments to do their own work. Again, if you're noticing sensations of resistance, I encourage you to be curious about why that might be.

That being said, my most sincere suggestion for healing companions is to ask the survivors in their care how they would like to be supported during their *body rites* healing journey. There's nothing like the feeling of having someone walk beside you while you're in it. Presence alone is often enough. And while *body rites* was created for Black survivors, experiences of violation, betrayal, and disembodiment are not unique to them. In this way, it may also be helpful to take the *body rites* journey yourself. The medicine is there for you. You deserve to be at home in your body too.

Trust your intuition—I talk about this relentlessly.

Most importantly, in holding them, *trust theirs*.

How can you as a healing companion nourish survivors' relationships with their intuition? This is the sweet spot.

I want to share my deepest gratitude for you and the care you offer in your embrace and space you hold. You're invited to consider the following prompts to guide you as a healing companion to your beloved survivors.

What does it mean to you to hold space?

Who are you in holding space? What is important to be mindful of?

How do you want survivors you hold space for to feel in your care?

I've offered some additional notes of inspiration for supporting Black survivors as healing companions to follow.

- Take a moment to celebrate your choice to be here. You might call into your awareness beloved survivors you've knowingly shared space with, and maybe even those you've unknowingly encountered.

- You're encouraged to ask your ego to take a back seat or a long nap. You might thank it for all the ways it keeps you safe and bolsters your confidence, and then offer it a place to observe and bear witness.

- Search for the parallels: the myriad manner that our stories, healing process, needs, places of struggle/resistance exist in tandem with the people we hold space for. You're encouraged to search for the moments when what you are reading also resonates with you, how the things a beloved survivor shares with you tug at something that lives within you, and perhaps how some of the tools strung throughout seem to change something for you.

- Hold separate space for yourself.

- Lean into your own support squads, support systems, and self care plans.

- Invite survivors to share what supporting them means or to share their self care plan with you.

- You're urgently encouraged to make the journey yourself. You might consider committing to the embodied healing journey in the workbook as an offering to your body and as a gesture of solidarity with survivors.

- Write in the margins, draw in the spaces provided, decorate the pages with your insights.

- Be willing to recall the times you messed up and to identify the approaches that are no longer aligned with being a space holder.

- Notice when after reading/reflecting you feel inspired and empowered to try something new in service of beloved survivors.

- Many mental health professionals trained from the western psychology lens have been unintentionally perpetuating harm by rooting therapeutic practices in Eurocentric values as the standard; by unknowingly perpetuating appropriation of ancient Indigenous healing wisdoms reupholstered as new-age psychological theory; and unconsciously furthering the agenda of colonization, patriarchy, and white supremacy in the space we hold. There is a lot to reconcile. I invite you to consider and actualize intentions to decolonize healing and therapy, urgently.

- If you are a mental health professional/healing practitioner, you might consider coplanning sessions with survivors guided by their respective healing journeys, spending as much time as feels right with each.

- There's no hurry. Healing takes time. Integration takes time.

- If you're a family member, friend, or loved one of a survivor, it might be helpful to coread *body rites*, noticing what stands out and sharing how you're available for support as you gain confidence.

- It may feel right to choose sections to explore together as home (body) work individually, in group formats, or as a team (you and survivor).

- Help survivors identify the choices/options available to them in any given moment.

- Respect their boundaries. Make asking them what their body is telling them a ritual in moments they are needing support. Over time, it'll become second nature.

- Stay within your scope, dear ones! There's a difference between supporting and therapy. Please respect the fine lines and encourage beloveds to seek professional services when it makes sense. We risk further harm when we operate outside of our lanes and skillsets.

Survivors heal themselves. They need you
to know and be with them in this truth.

acknowledgments | modúpẹ*

Black beings at home in their bodies are forces of nature.

and navigating the elements with survivors is the sacred work that feels most natural to me. thank you for trusting me to hold you in these pages.

as I wrote this book, I realized it was an inevitable thing. I found solace in writing and dancing as a little girl. writing was a vault to capture the feelings and stories that trauma would otherwise bury in places I have yet to find. dance and movement relentlessly pulled me back into my body. these were the seeds that blossomed my own healing journey. I discovered yoga in 2008 and it changed my life. I stretched out into myself. I felt all the things. my spiritual senses heightened. the quiet space in my mind was luminous and ripe for insight and deeper awareness. I am deeply grateful for the ancient medicine that is yoga, how easily it forgives, and how eagerly it awaits my return when I drift.

body rites began with a nudge in the early morning hours, "write this down" they said. a couple of weeks later, while journeying Mexico's Yucatan state, I was on a call with Deborah, who would become my editor at Norton. the spirit of this book knew when it wanted to come into this world and writing it has been one of the most holy moments of my lifetime.

there are many people, places, and energies to thank.

thank you Zabie-boo for being the exception in so many ways. I love healing and holding in tandem with you. you are the god–mother of this book.

modúpẹ to dr. Thema for your push, and the willingness to speak into my ear on being and on bossing.

to the most special lands of the Mayab (Yucatan, Mexico) for being a safe place to dream about this book. my sweetest gratitude to my dear friend Solana who somehow lives up to her name even on cloudy days—you were the first to know and the first to celebrate with me. Xaymaca (Portland, Jamaica) you changed me. thank you for embracing me and cocooning me in your plush mountains, for restoring me in your cool waters, for the night songs of the peene walis that became my writing soundtrack, and for your magical people. Queen Nanny power to all of you.

modúpẹ to my body for its enduring ability to experience and alchemize, for being my griot, and my voice when I didn't have the words. thank you for being one of the authors of this book. modúpẹ to the healing practices that have kept me and cared for me—yoga, modern and West African dance. to little shena, thank you for teaching me self-compassion, how to love in spite of, and for holding onto your most sweet essence.

I give thanks to the best in my family members, survivors, and ancestor–survivors within my bloodlines. may you experience redemption and vicarious healing in my creating this book.

---

* modúpẹ translates to I give thanks in Yoruba, mojúbà translates to I give respect.

may it touch us all and our generations forward. may our blood and cells one day be free of any remnants of sexual violation.

to my chosen family, closest beloveds, friends, and loves, there is not enough empty space to capture the home you have created for me in your collective embrace and in the many moments you have stood in the gaps. to my little Zoe—you made so many of my days and stole my heart. modúpẹ́ to my spiritual family Baba Fasegun, Iya Fayomi, my Ibeji community in Los Angeles and across the waters in Ode Remo and Ibadan, Nigeria.

modúpẹ́ and rivers of respect to Chante DeLoach and all of my teachers, sacred texts I've held close, to any healing-practitioner/therapist that has held space for me. I have *become* in your presence, gaze, and wisdom.

gratitude beams from my heart to the *embodied truth healing* community—to my clients past, present, and future, I love you (and all the parts of you). thank you for the gift exchanges of our time together and for trusting me.

bottomless thank yous to my editor Deborah Malmud, Mariah Eppes, and the Norton team. you all truly gave me the room and pen to write the book I dreamed of. thank you for understanding that being author and artist are one and the same for me.

modúpẹ́ to the beautiful ones who chose to be muses for the alchemizing art series throughout the book—Ullanda Davis, London Jones, Ahmunet Jordon, Brandy El Sayed, kiyama monique, Nityda Bhakti Gessel, Alishia McCullough, Aunjel Fullington, Mckenna Anderson, and Iya Osunkeye Katrice Jackson. I hope that you will continue to remember the power in choosing where to put your yeses. radiating gratitude to my beloved teachers Iya Fayomi and xochi for placing your prayers here, for codivining with me, and for your sincerest excitement!

my dearest shyma, you are a wonder I am so fortunate to know. I would not have wanted to do this with anyone else. your art is always an opportunity to be moved. your friendship lives in me as though we've known each other since we were littles. thanks for opening to my love so long ago. I love you. I am happy you exist. #G4L

To the second author(s) of this book—may you be pleased with your work. it is my most profound honor to be the channel from your lips to these pages. I am enamored by your poeticism, nuanced power, and majesty.

modúpẹ́ Ori, you are the blessing.

mojúbà Orunmila, Olodumare, Ifa.

ore YeYeooo, ibà àṣẹ.

references |

Afedefeyo, I. O. (2017). The white book. Distributed by Ile Orunmila Afedefeyo.

Arewa, C. S. (1998). *Opening to Spirit: Contacting the healing power of the chakras & honouring African spirituality*. Afrikan World Books.

Beattie, M. (2009). *The new codependency: Help and guidance for today's generation*. Simon & Schuster Paperbacks: New York, NY.

Bird, S. R. (2009). *A healing grove: African tree remedies and rituals for the body and spirit*. Chicago Review Press.

Brownmiller, S. (1975). *Against our will: Men, women, and rape*. New York: Fawcett Books.

Campbell, R., Self, T., & Ahrens, C.E. (2003). The physical health consequences of rape: Assessing survivors' somatic symptoms in a racially diverse population. *Women's Studies Quarterly, 31*(1/2), 99–104.

Collins, P. H. (2000). *Black feminist thought: Knowledge, consciousness, and the politics of empowerment*. New York: Routledge.

Damasio, A.R. (2000). *The feeling of what happens: Body and emotion in the making of consciousness*. Random House; New York.

Dana, D. (2021). *Anchored: How to befriend your nervous system using polyvagal theory*. Sounds True: Boulder, CO.

DeGruy, J. (2017). *Post traumatic slave syndrome: America's legacy of enduring injury and healing*. Joy DeGruy Publications Inc.

Duraiswamy, G., Thirthalli, J., Nagendra, H.R., & Gangadhar, B.N. (2007). Yoga therapy as an add-on treatment in the management of patients with schizophrenia: A randomized controlled trial. *Acta Psychiatrica Scandinavica, 116*(3), 226–232. doi: 10.1111/j.1600-0447.2007.01032.x

Eden, D. & Feinstein, D. (2008). *Energy medicine: Balancing your body's energies for optimal health, joy, and vitality*. Penguin Random House.

Emerson, D. & Hopper, E. (2011). *Overcoming trauma through yoga: Reclaiming your body*. North Atlantic Books: Berkeley, CA.

Hall, J. (1983). The mind that burns in each body: Women, rape, and racial violence. In A. Snitow, C. Stansell, & S. Thompson (Eds.), *Powers of desire: The politics of sexuality* (pp. 328, 332–33). Monthly Review Press: New York.

James, S. E., Herman, J. L., Rankin, S., Keisling, M., Mottet, L., & Anafi, M. (2016). *The report of the 2015 U.S. transgender survey*. National Center for Transgender Equality: Washington, DC.

Karade, B. I. (1994). *The handbook of Yoruba religious concepts*. Weiser Books: Boston, MA/York Beach, ME.

Kemetic Yoga Association. (n.d.). Retrieved from http://www.kemeticyoga.org/what_is_kemetic_yoga_.

Mbiti, J. S. (1975). *Introduction to African religion*. Heinemann Educational: London.

Menakem, R. (2017). *My grandmother's hands*. Central Recovery Press.

National Sexual Violence Resource Center. (2013). *Building cultures of care: A guide for sexual assault services programs*. https://www.nsvrc.org/sites/default/files/2017-10/publications_nsvrc_building-cultures-of-care.pdf

Roberts, D. (1998). *Killing the Black body: Race, reproduction, and the meaning of liberty*. New York: Vintage.

Ross, A. & Thomas, S. (2010). The health benefits of yoga and exercise: A review of comparison studies. *The Journal of Alternative and Complementary Medicine, 16*(1), 3–12. doi: 10.1089/acm.2009.0044.

Rothschild, B. (2000). *The body remembers: The psychosociology of trauma and trauma treatment*. Norton.

Sawandi, T. (n.d.). *Yorubic Medicine: The art of divine herbology*. Partnering with plants ebook.

Segal, I. (2010). *The secret language of your body: The essential guide to health and wellness.* Beyond Words.

Shapiro, D., Cook, I. A., Davydov, D. M., Ottaviani, C., Leuchter, A. F., & Abrams, M. (2007). Yoga as a complementary treatment of depression: Effects of traits and moods on treatment outcome. *Evidence Based Complementary Alternative Medicine, 4,* 493–502. doi: 10.1093/ecam/nel114.

Siegel, D. J. (2012). *The developing mind: How relationships and the brain interact to shape who we are* (2nd ed.). The Guilford Press: NY.

Scott, T. (n.d.). An African herbalist's overview of partnering with plants- ebookStanford Encyclopedia of Philosophy. (2011). *Feminist perspectives on objectification.* Retrieved from http://plato.stanford.edu/entries/feminism-objectification/.

Teish, L. (1985). *Jambalaya: The natural woman's book of personal charms and practical rituals.* Harper One.

The National Center on Violence Against Women in the Black Community. (October 2018). *Black women and sexual assault.* https://ujimacommunity.org/wp-content/uploads/2018/12/Ujima-Womens-Violence-Stats-v7.4-1.pdf

Tjaden, P. & Thoenness, N. (2000). *Prevalence, incidence, and consequences of violence against women: Findings from the national violence against women survey.* U.S. Department of Justice: National Institute of Justice Centers for Disease Control and Prevention.

Planty, M., Langton, L., Krebs, C., Berzofsky, M., & Smiley-McDonald, H. (2013). *Female victims of sexual violence, 1994-2010.* U.S. Department of Justice Statistics. https://bjs.ojp.gov/content/pub/pdf/fvsv9410.pdf

van der Kolk, B. (2014). *The body keeps the score: Brain, mind and body in the healing of trauma.* Penguin Publishing Group.

Woodruff, D. (n.d.). How to make an herb-infused oil. In *Partnering with plants* (pp. 91–94). [Ebook].

Wyatt, G. E. (1992). The sociocultural context of African American and White American women's rape. *Journal of Social Issues, 48*(1), 77–91.

xóchicoatl. (2021). la mala yerba herbal action glossary.

Yamasaki, Z. (2022) *trauma-informed yoga for survivors of sexual assault practices for healing and teaching with compassion.* New York: Norton.

index |

index

about the author | dr. shena j young

dr. shena j young (she/her) is a licensed body centered psychologist–healer, artist, and Iyalorisa of Osun and Obatala in the Isese tradition of Ifa. affectionately known as dr. shena, she intimately works with folks of the global majority, anchored in the pillars of remembrance, sovereignty, authenticity, intuition, and self-determination. she holds space internationally for individuals, couples, groups, and organizations committed to the ritual of calling themselves back into their bodies as a freedom practice. she owns a private practice, *embodied truth healing & psychological services*, rooted in Los Angeles, CA where she offers mind–body–heart–spirit care in healing from sexual, racial, intergenerational, and ancestral traumas. in community, she intuitively designs holistic moments of healing that embrace the whole person and beloved communities as they are.

her approach to healing divests from the westernized blueprint, as it traverses the body, land-based approaches and connection with nature, and indigenous wisdoms and African spiritual traditions as the medicine. healing with dr. shena is a visceral experience that evokes and people trust her, because in space with her they remember how to trust themselves.

dr. shena's voice has been featured in *Bustle, Huffington Post, Lily by The Washington Post, Therapy for Black Girls*, and she has been trusted to care and consult for *The Body: A Home for Love, Black Girl in OM, Loveland Foundation, and metoo movement* communities among many others.

@embodiedtruthhealing

about the illustrator | dr. shyma el sayed

shyma el sayed (she/her) is an artist, psychologist, and healer who loves exploring new mediums of expression. trained in the fine arts in nyc, the past few years she has expanded her exploration to include digital art. in the *body rites* series, she interweaves her love for traditional mediums, emotive styles, and the modern simplicity of digital design. she credits her inspiration to be the beauty and strength that emanate from all womxn survivors, working to capture the diversity of the individual while also reflecting the divinity of the collective. to each of the travelers on their sacred journey, shyma has this to say, *may you find your own alchemy reflected in these pages knowing that you are seen, accepted, and most of all loved.*

this body of work is dedicated to my Moonberries, whose guiding light will forever shine in her four stars.

about the contributors |

Trifari Williams (she/her), aka Iya Fayomi Osundoyin Egbeyemi, has been a practitioner of African Traditional Religion (ATR) her entire life. As a young girl she studied under the tutelage of Iya Luisa Teish. In the spring of 2007 the Oba, Awo Bolu Fatunmise, initiated her into the mysteries of Ifa. One year after her first initiation she became a Priestess of Osun in the epicenter of Ifa Tradition, Ile Ife, Nigeria. Most recently she was initiated into Egbe and Kori, in Ode Remo, focusing her priesthood on the healing work of women, and fertility. She currently serves as Head Priestess and provides spiritual counsel to the Ifa community through her Spiritual House, Ile Orunmila Afedefeyo, in Los Angeles, CA. Trifari was born to a Chicana mother and an African (American) father, who raised her to be firmly rooted in her ancestral traditions. As a woman who identifies as African-Mexican she has seen the world through a lens that is deeply rooted in rich culture and also makes her acutely aware of the Black and brown experience in the United States.

xóchicoatl bello (they/she/amor) is an indigequeer healing practitioner, cultural worker, educator, earth steward, and elder-in-training. They come from Afro-indigenous, Portuguese, and Spanish bloods via love and colonization rooted in Southern Mexico, from a people recovering their memory, from a people in treaties with peoples and lands alike reclaiming their sovereignty. xóchicoatl focuses on cultivating cultures of healing by restoring our connections to the sacredness of self, each other, earth, and ancestor through ceremony, circle practice, indigenous technologies and agricultural traditions. They hold healing spaces in relationship with the Earth with the prayer that when we heal the soils that sustain us, tend to the seeds, tend to our hearts, and tend to our relations, we remember our bodies as sites of wisdom, we heal our souls, and we awaken ancestral memory that we have always been free. to connect with their work visit lamalayerba.com, to be in relationship with their sweet prayers weave with them on instagram.com @lamalayerbalove.